QUICK GUIDES

Post-natal Health

LIZ EARLE'S
QUICK GUIDES

Post-natal Health

B⬛XTREE

Advice to the Reader
Before following any dietary advice contained in this book, it is recommended that you consult your doctor if you suffer from any health problems or special condition or are in any doubt.

First published in Great Britain in 1995 by Boxtree Limited,
Broadwall House, 21 Broadwall, London SE1 9PL

Copyright © Liz Earle 1995
All rights reserved

The right of Liz Earle to be identified as Author of this Work has been asserted by her in accordance with the Copyright, Designs and Patents Act 1988

10 9 8 7 6 5 4 3 2 1

ISBN: 0 7522 1690 2

Text design by Blackjacks
Cover design by Hammond Hammond

Except in the United States of America this book is sold subject to the condition that it shall not, by way of trade or otherwise, be lent, resold, hired out or otherwise circulated without the publisher's prior consent in any form of binding or cover than that in which it is published and without a similar condition including this condition being imposed upon a subsequent purchaser

Printed and Bound in Great Britain by Cox & Wyman Ltd.,
Reading, Berkshire

A CIP catalogue entry for this book is available from
the British Library

Contents

Acknowledgements 6

Introduction 7

1 The First Few Weeks 9

2 Natural Remedies for Common Problems 23

3 Breastfeeding and Beyond 33

4 The Baby Blues 51

5 Getting Back into Shape 61

6 Natural Baby Care 77

Glossary 89

Useful Addresses 91

Index 93

ACKNOWLEDGEMENTS

I am grateful to Carla Smith for helping to produce this book. I am also indebted to the talented team at Boxtree and to Rosemary Sandberg and Claire Bowles Publicity for their unfailing enthusiasm and support.

Introduction

Having a baby changes your life – not only the practical aspect of becoming somebody's parent, but also on many mental, emotional and physical levels. As the mother of two children, I am keenly aware of how it feels to have just given birth. I have also personally experienced many of the highs and lows of early parenthood. This *Quick Guide* aims to make every woman's transition to motherhood as enjoyable and effortless as possible. I wish you a lifetime of joy and happiness with your new offspring – and hope that my *Quick Guide to Post-natal Health* will help you in the first few months of this long and eventful journey of life.

Liz Earle

1

The First Few Weeks

Congratulations – You've Just Had a Baby!

Giving birth is one of the most miraculous and unique experiences in life. Whether you have had a thrilling and satisfying birth or a long and painful one, you now begin a new role in life. After carrying your baby during the months of your pregnancy, at last you meet him or her and begin the exciting transition to parenthood.

It may take a while to appreciate that you have actually become a parent. You are now responsible for a small baby – something you may not have experienced before. You are to clothe, feed and care for a tiny human being, who is totally dependent on you. This is completely different to being pregnant, when the baby was developing in your womb leaving you with plenty of time to do exactly what you wanted. You now have a full-time commitment to your new child and all the demands on your time and energy that come with him or her.

The first few days after giving birth can be a tiring but thrilling time for you and your partner. This miraculous event may leave you both on a high for a couple of days as you feel the intense pleasure that comes from creating and producing a new human being. You may look at your baby with wonder and not quite believe that your pregnancy has culminated in this tiny, needy creature. You may also feel great pride in your achievement and the fact you have started a new life with very little help from anyone else!

POST-NATAL HEALTH

Your Emotions

When you've come down to earth after giving birth you may begin to experience a wide range of feelings. While having a baby is a unique experience, it can be highly emotional and sometimes exhausting. You may be feeling elated, weepy, anxious – or just completely exhausted. Emotions run high after you've given birth, so don't be surprised if your moods swing from high to low in a short period of time.

Be prepared for a degree of shock, too. Not only do you have to deal with the emotional side of having a new baby, you may be suffering from a range of physical side-effects – both from having given birth and from your body's adapting to no longer being pregnant. Plus, if you've had a Caesarean delivery or stitches, it will take your body a while to return to normal.

You may also feel very tired and need plenty of rest and support from family and friends. This is the time to spoil yourself and to let other people cook you meals and help out with the housework. Don't worry about the dust – just concentrate on yourself and your new baby. Try to limit your visitors to just a couple each day and ask them if they'd mind making it short. It's vital that you and your partner have plenty of time to yourselves – so you can get to know your baby and adjust to your new lifestyle.

Try to relax and enjoy these first few weeks with your newborn. It's not always easy to stay calm with a brand new baby – particularly if he or she is your first – but, in the long term, staying relaxed will help you get used to your new situation and enable you to recover more quickly. Savour these special moments with your baby – you'll never be able to repeat them!

THE FIRST FEW WEEKS

Your Body

It should take about six weeks for your body to return to its pre-pregnant state – perhaps a little longer if you have had a difficult birth. During these first few weeks, it's vital that you try to relax as much as possible, take gentle exercise such as walking and eat a healthy, well-balanced diet. Looking after yourself, as well as your baby, will enable you to adjust to your baby's birth quickly and ensure you stay fit and healthy.

After the birth, your uterus continues to contract until it reaches its former size. As a result, you may feel mild period-like cramps or have stronger, more uncomfortable pains. With your first baby, you will probably feel very little, but the afterpains do get worse with each subsequent birth as your uterus has to work harder to contract back to its previous size. This pain can be worse when you are breastfeeding, as the baby's sucking action can encourage the womb to contract. Although uncomfortable, this helps your body to get back into shape more quickly.

The pressure of the baby's head coming down your birth canal may leave you feeling a little uncomfortable and swollen for a couple of weeks. If your perineum tore or you had a cut (episiotomy), you will feel more pain – but even if you had neither you may still suffer slight bruises and grazes which will heal naturally. Taking the homoeopathic Arnica 30C tablets every four hours can significantly speed the healing process and reduce bruising. If the birth was particularly quick or you had to push very hard for a long time you may feel uncomfortable.

When you pass water, you may feel a stinging or burning sensation in your vaginal area. Instead of the toilet, it may be easier to use a bidet, or use a shower, running water between your legs while you urinate. Another way to ease this problem is to keep a bottle or jug filled with cold water next to the toilet and to pour it between your legs each time you empty your bladder. Instead of drying yourself with toilet paper you may prefer to use a hairdryer (on a cool setting) for the first day or so!

Immediately after the birth you will lose blood and will experience a discharge, called lochia, from your vagina. At first this may be quite heavy – so make sure you have some super-thick sanitary pads handy – but don't use tampons as they can cause infection in the first few weeks after the birth. Your midwife will check this regularly as heavy bleeding may lead to anaemia. If there are large clots or an unpleasant-smelling discharge, you may have a uterine infection. If you experience these, or are bleeding excessively, do consult your doctor or midwife.

Lochia is bright red during the first few days after the birth and then turns reddish brown for a while before becoming brown and ceasing. It can last up to six weeks. Don't worry if it turns red again for a few days after you have got up from your bed rest or if it restarts when you thought it had stopped. This is quite normal.

Recovering from a Difficult Birth

Some women, particularly first-time mothers, feel physically exhausted and battered after giving birth. This may be because there had to be a great deal of obstetric intervention – either because the baby was lying in a difficult position, or perhaps your physical structure was too small for the baby's easy passage through the birth canal. The labour might have had to be induced, because you were past your due date, or your contractions may have been accelerated with drugs. This may have made the contractions very fast and painful, making you feel tired and weak after the birth. In addition, you might have suffered torn muscles and ligaments, and experienced more bruising and bleeding than a woman who had an easier birth.

THE FIRST FEW WEEKS

If you did have a demanding and exhausting birth, you may feel that it's you who needs plenty of care and attention – not just your baby. Try these tips to relax and gently bring yourself back to health:

* If you don't have the energy to get out of bed, try to do some simple movements while lying down. Start by rotating your ankles and sliding your feet up and down the bed. Try doing a few pelvic floor exercises (see Chapter 5).
* You may be suffering a lot of pain because of stitches, but do try to pass water regularly. If it's too painful to sit on the toilet, just stand above it while you urinate.
* Drink as much as possible. This will prevent you from getting constipation, which hurts a sore perineum. If you do get constipation, ask for some glycerine suppositories. Alternatively, swallow a handful of linseeds with a large glass of water. This is an excellent natural remedy for constipation. You probably won't empty your bowels until two or three days after giving birth.
* Try to relax. Get out of bed and have a couple of warm baths each day. Put a couple of drops of your favourite essential oil in the bath water to help you unwind. Good choices include lavender and sandalwood. Breathe deeply and perhaps play some soothing music as you soak.
* Make sure you have plenty of help during the first couple of weeks at home – to look after your baby and do some housework. Take up every offer from grandparents, friends and neighbours!
* If you feel you were not treated well and your demands were not taken into consideration during the birth, write a letter of complaint to the hospital management.

POST-NATAL HEALTH

This will not only make you feel better by getting it off your chest, but may improve the system for future mums-to-be.

Coping after a Caesarean Birth

It can take about six months to recover from a Caesarean birth. But, as in a vaginal birth, you will experience the same changes to your uterus and have the same discharges. You may feel an itching sensation as the wound heals – and will find when your pubic hair regrows that your scar is almost completely hidden.

It may be the last thing you want to do, but a little gentle exercise is very important if you've had a Caesarean. Start with your feet while you're still in bed – just move them in small circles – this will get the circulation going in your legs. When you can do more exercise, try pelvic tilting and pelvic rocking (see Chapter 5). This will help to tone up the muscles which were cut through in the operation. The most important factor is to avoid lifting anything remotely heavy.

When you're breastfeeding your baby after a Caesarean, you can either lie on your side, with the baby next to you, or put the baby on your lap, with her legs under one arm and use the other hand to bring the baby's head to your breast (placing your baby on a cushion may make this easier).

Your Breasts

After your baby is born, your breasts will appear very much larger. If you decide not to breastfeed, you will be prescribed medication to suppress the normal milk production and your breasts will return to their normal size about a week later. But if you are breastfeeding, it is worth investing in a couple of

THE FIRST FEW WEEKS

nursing bras, which make feeding simpler. These usually come with clips or zips attached to the cups – so you don't have to take the bra off to feed and give your baby easy access to the breast.

For the first few days after the birth, your breasts secrete a special food called colostrum. This yellowish liquid contains all the antibodies your baby needs to protect him or her from illness and disease. It is richer in protein than your later milk and helps the baby to sleep for long periods between feeds. This may be nature's way of giving you a rest after a tiring birth! Even if you do not intend to breastfeed, it is well worth giving your baby this very special elixir as it is a nutritious start to life.

If your baby sucks on the colostrum, your milk will come in between the second and the sixth day after you've given birth. When this happens you may experience the 'let-down reflex'. This is a warm tingling or 'pins and needles' sensation created by hormones which have flowed into the blood vessels in your breasts, causing cells around your milk glands to contract, squeezing milk out through the holes in your nipples. Not all women feel this – so don't worry if you don't feel the let-down reflex – your milk will still be there for your baby.

When your milk arrives, your breasts will probably feel very full and you may even have the sensation that you're about to burst. This fullness is called engorgement and usually disappears in a couple of days. If your breasts are engorged, feed your baby frequently as it's important to empty the breasts and relieve this feeling. A warm bath or shower followed by a feed may help to reduce engorgement. Also, try placing very hot flannels around the breasts and use gentle massage strokes to help clear blocked milk ducts.

The milk produced by your breasts looks thinner than the colostrum. The fore milk, which your baby has at the start of the feed is thirst quenching and gives your baby a drink before the richer hind milk, which is the main meal of the feed.

Your breasts may leak for the first few days after your milk has come in, so try wearing breast pads inside your bra to soak up any runaway droplets. The amount of milk you produce will gradually regulate itself according to the quantity needed by your baby and you will lose the uncomfortable full feeling.

If you are breastfeeding you might not restart your periods until you stop feeding, or for a few weeks or months after that. If you aren't breastfeeding, menstruation might begin as early as a month after the birth. But it could also begin later. It's worth thinking about contraception as soon as possible as you can become pregnant before your periods start again. Breastfeeding is *not* an effective form of contraception, and you could end up with two babies less than a year apart – it has been known!

Your New Shape

After the birth, you may feel incredibly light and sylph-like – having lost the weight of the baby, the placenta and water. But you may be a little surprised that you don't immediately return to your pre-pregnant shape. Your tummy will probably look a little saggy after giving birth and, despite having lost the weight of the baby, the placenta and a lot of fluid, you may still be quite a lot larger than you were before you became pregnant. This is partly because your muscles have stretched. However, if you eat a balanced diet and start doing some gentle exercise such as pelvic tilts and abdominal curls (see Chapter 5), your pre-pregnancy figure should return.

Your stomach muscles will have stretched to accommodate your growing uterus and this may have produced a dark line running down the middle of your abdomen – the linea negra. This should disappear soon after the birth so don't panic about it.

Hair Loss

You may also be surprised to find that your hair begins to fall out after you've had your baby. It may fall out in handfuls or you'll simply find a lot in your hairbrush after brushing. Don't worry – this is very common after pregnancy and is caused by changing hormone levels and, possibly, nutritional deficiencies. Basically, your body hangs on to hair during pregnancy so, when you've had the baby, you may lose nine months' worth in one go. Make sure you are looking after yourself with a healthy diet which includes plenty of protein and vitamin B (essential for healthy hair). Try also to avoid drinking coffee and alcohol as they can reduce your stores of B vitamins.

Think about getting your hair cut in an easy and manageable style and wash it with a mild shampoo. Treating yourself to a new hair style can give you a real boost and renewed confidence.

Continued Care

The first few days with your baby will be exhausting but rewarding. You will need to recover your strength from the birth so, if you leave hospital early, do make sure there's someone around to do the shopping, washing, cooking and household chores for you in the early days. You need all the rest you can get – so ask a friend or relative if they'd mind dropping in once a day to help out.

If you leave hospital before the baby is ten days old or have had a home birth, a community midwife will visit you every day to make sure everything is fine and to help you care for your baby. She will also make sure you are shaping up physically by checking up on your breasts, uterus and any stitches you have had. If you are finding breastfeeding difficult, she can help you

POST-NATAL HEALTH

with this and suggest new feeding positions. If you have any worries about yourself or the baby make sure you mention them to your midwife.

Ten days after the birth, the health visitor takes over from the midwife. She is a trained nurse who cares for the emotional and physical health of mother and baby. She will visit you once or twice to weigh the baby and, if all is well, you can then take your baby to see her at the local clinic once a week.

POST-NATAL CHECK-UP

Your doctor or obstetrician will wish to see you about six weeks after the birth to give you a complete post-natal check-up, as follows:

* Your blood pressure will be checked.
* Your breasts may be examined.
* You will be given an internal examination to see if your pelvic floor muscles are well toned and if the uterus and bladder are in the correct position.
* Any scar tissue or stitches resulting from the birth will also be checked.
* A cervical smear may be taken.
* The doctor will ask if you still have any vaginal discharge and if you have had a period.
* You will probably be asked about any contraception needs.

The six-week check-up is a good opportunity to discuss any worries with your doctor. If you are having any problems such as unhealed stitches or painful sex, do mention them. Before you go in, scribble down any questions or worries you have about your health. Do be honest with your doctor – make sure you have the opportunity to discuss your problems with him or her face to face – not while you are lying on your back during an

THE FIRST FEW WEEKS

examination. Don't be afraid to ask for help – especially if you are feeling very low or depressed or if you are worried.

Starting Sex

Returning to your previous sex life may not happen immediately – you may feel apprehensive, particularly if you've had stitches. You may not want to have sex for several weeks, or even months, especially after a long and traumatic birth. Some women prefer to wait until after their six-week check-up, when they know all is well, before they make love again.

If you are at all nervous, the best way to approach sex is gently. Don't necessarily rush into full intercourse immediately. Choose a quiet time when your baby is asleep, and slowly rediscover your partner's body. Try giving each other a gentle massage, just to get used to each other again. After a few of these cuddling sessions you may feel ready for sex. Use a lubricant if your vagina is feeling dry (this is common in the early weeks) and ask your partner to be slow and gentle.

If penetration hurts because you've had an episiotomy, try different ways of lovemaking for a while, until sex is easier. If it is still painful a couple of months after the birth, go and see your doctor for a check-up.

Arrange your method of contraception as soon as possible. You can become pregnant again soon after the birth of your baby, even if you are breastfeeding and even if you haven't restarted your periods.

Baby Blues

You may feel on a complete high immediately after giving birth, and find it difficult to sleep for the first couple of nights.

POST-NATAL HEALTH

You might want to gaze in wonder at your baby rather than dropping off to sleep! This elation may give way to feeling very weepy between the third and fifth day after you've had the baby. You may worry about small problems or frequently burst into tears. This is quite normal as your body and emotions have been through a huge upheaval and you're bound to want to cry a little.

Baby blues can be caused by fatigue, changes in your hormones, pain from stitches or sore breasts or simply from a feeling of anticlimax after the build-up to the birth. You may just need some rest or a good cry. Talk about your feelings to your partner, friends or midwife. The baby blues should only last for a day or two – if it lasts for longer or becomes more of a depression, seek help as soon as possible, (see Chapter 4).

Your Diet

If you were eating healthily during your pregnancy there is no need to stop now. Eat as much fresh food as you can, with plenty of fruit and vegetables. To boost your energy levels and help you cope with the demands of a new baby, eat lots of unrefined carbohydrates and fibre, such as potatoes, wholewheat bread, pasta, brown rice and beans. This will also help you avoid constipation and return your bowels back to normal after the birth. If you are still straining when you wish to empty your bowels, add more fibre-rich fruits and vegetables to your meals and try taking linseeds with water between meals.

Eating plenty of protein is also important to help you repair any tissues damaged during the birth and to help you produce breastmilk. Choose from dairy products, any kind of beans and pulses (such as lentils and chickpeas), fish, seafood and meat products for your protein intake. Try also to eat food with a high iron content such as red meat, green vegetables and dried fruit – especially if you're feeling tired and washed out after the birth. You may also like to consider a supplementary liquid or iron tonic, such as the excellent Floravital.

You may have put on some weight during your pregnancy, but this is not a good time to diet – especially if you are breastfeeding. Try to avoid fatty, convenience and sweet foods and if you feel you must have a treat, make it a healthy one, such as a bowl of yoghurt, honey and banana, or a wholefood health bar.

When preparing food, try to go for simple recipes which don't need pre-planning or complicated ingredients. Then you can simply rush into the kitchen and knock up a meal without taking too much time or trouble. Better still, ask your partner to take over the cooking.

EXTRA ESSENTIALS

Research has shown that lack of vitamin B and calcium can contribute to post-natal depression – so it's worth taking these as supplements to try and prevent the problem. If you're feeling at all irritable, moody and emotional, you may be lacking the B vitamins. So either buy a good B-complex vitamin supplement or eat more wholegrains and animal protein.

As you lose blood in the first couple of weeks after the birth – lowering your haemoglobin levels – it's worth taking an iron supplement. To help your body absorb iron, try eating a lot of vitamin C-rich foods – such as citrus fruits, broccoli, potatoes and cabbage. If you've had a particularly long and tiring birth you may be prescribed iron tablets; however, these often cause constipation.

If you're breastfeeding it is worth taking a zinc supplement as you need plenty of the mineral during this time. One study found that the zinc content of food eaten by pregnant and breastfeeding women was only 42 percent of the recommended daily allowance. A good daily intake is 15–20mg (make sure you take the elemental as opposed to the compound zinc). Try to avoid drinking coffee after taking zinc as this can halve the amount you actually absorb.

When breastfeeding you may be short of folic acid – vital for normal cell function and the production of red blood cells. You can either buy a supplement or find it in dry beans and fresh green vegetables such as spinach and lettuce. You will absorb folic acid more easily if you eat plenty of foods rich in vitamins C and B. Bear in mind that your need for vitamins and minerals increases during breastfeeding, so a well-balanced multivitamin and mineral formula would be worth taking.

You and Your Partner

Having a baby is bound to alter the relationship you have with your partner. Your new child not only means a fundamental change to your life, but also to that of your husband or boyfriend. You now have an extra responsibility, coupled with less freedom than you both enjoyed before. This can lead to arguments and perhaps a feeling of entrapment – on either side. That's why it is very important for you both to talk about the way you feel about your changed life and your new baby. If you find you are arguing more in the early weeks – don't worry – you are probably both very tired with little time for each other or yourselves. Sometimes just getting a little more sleep or having a couple of hours alone together without the baby can help.

You must also consider the feelings of any other children in your family who may be jealous of this new arrival who takes up so much of your time. Reassure them that your new baby will not change the love you have for them.

——2——
Natural Remedies for Common Problems

You may be on a wonderful natural high after giving birth, but be irritated by minor problems such as discomfort from stitches or piles. Don't worry – many women experience these problems during the first few weeks after giving birth. Try using natural therapies such as homoeopathy or aromatherapy to ease any small ailments you may have at this time. If you're feeling tired or stressed you can also find natural ways to help you to rest and relax.

Aromatherapy

This soothing therapy uses fragrant and powerful essential oils, extracted from flowers, trees and herbs, to treat a wide range of physical and mental problems. Treatment of the whole human being – incorporating body, mind and mood – is very important as the physical body and the mind are closely linked.

Aromatherapy works through your sense of smell and via absorption into the skin. Our sense of smell has a profound and immediate effect on the way we feel – probably because smells access the brain directly – particularly the emotional part of the brain. Essential oils are easily absorbed by the skin because of their small molecular structure. They are quickly absorbed into the bloodstream and then travel throughout the body via an intricate network of blood vessels, which means they can work on the entire body.

The essential oils are too highly concentrated to be used neat on the skin – so for massage they should be mixed with a carrier or base oil such as almond, grapeseed or wheatgerm oil. Essential oils can be bought in health-food shops and by mail order from aromatherapy oil suppliers.

Homoeopathy

This is a natural medicine, created in the late eighteenth century by Samuel Hahnemann, a German doctor. Unlike conventional medicine, homoeopathy looks at physical symptoms as attempts by your body to expel disease. So a homoeopath will treat your illness by giving you a tiny dose of the same ailment, instead of prescribing a medicine to suppress the symptoms. So if you had a very sore throat, the homoeopath might give you a minute dose of a substance which causes sore throats in a healthy person. This makes the body fight back and release its own ability to heal.

When you visit a homoeopath, the treatment begins with a long assessment, with the practitioner asking questions about your emotional and physical history. This is because homoeopaths believe that people react differently to the same disease.

If you want to treat yourself, homoeopathic remedies are available in most health-food shops and chemists and come in the form of a soft pill or powder. Always follow these guidelines when treating yourself:

* Find a remedy which matches your personality and lifestyle – not just your symptoms.
* Avoid coffee and peppermint while taking homoeopathic remedies as they lessen the effectiveness of the treatment.

NATURAL REMEDIES FOR COMMON PROBLEMS

* Homoeopathic remedies come in various doses. The 6c, 12c and 30c are all safe to take at home. Don't go over 30c.
* Repeat the dosage according to the severity of your symptoms – every ten minutes if you feel terrible – and take the remedy less often if you begin to feel better. If you have taken six doses and there is no improvement, change the remedy or visit a homoeopath.

Natural Remedy Finder

BACK PAIN

You may experience some backache after giving birth. This is fairly common, as the pregnancy may have put stress on your back, or because of the lengthy straining and pushing during the second stage of labour. If you had an epidural, you may feel back pain at the point where the needle for the epidural was inserted.

Helping yourself

Make sure you are bending properly (see Chapter 5) when picking up your baby or doing the housework. You should always bend your knees when picking up any kind of weight. If you have muscular tension, try drinking soothing herbal teas such as chamomile and lemon balm. It may be worth visiting a cranial osteopath (especially if you had an epidural) to check the nerve fibres and cerebrospinal fluid around the spine.

Aromatherapy remedy

Ask your partner to massage your back with 50ml almond oil and ten drops of a mixture of any of the following essential oils: citrus, geranium, patchouli and sandalwood.

POST-NATAL HEALTH

Homoeopathy remedy
If your back feels weak and tired with dragging pains in the middle and lower back, take Kali carbonicum. Belladonna should be taken if your head feels hot and there is a hard, tense feeling in your lower abdomen. If you have this hard tense feeling and feel hot all over, take Pulsatilla. If you feel chilly and also have this hard, tense feeling in the lower abdomen, take Nux vomica. Other remedies to choose from are Arnica, Bryonia, Hypericum and Rhus toxicodendron.

STITCHES
Many women are given stitches after the birth because of a tear or a cut (episiotomy). These can feel uncomfortable for several days afterwards, especially when sitting down, passing urine or opening your bowels.

Helping yourself
* Gently bathing the area often helps stitches to heal – wash in a bath or bidet or just use cotton wool and warm water.
* Throwing a few handfuls of sea salt into your bath can also help stitches to heal. After washing, dry the area carefully.
* Get as much air to the area as possible – this also helps stitches to heal quicker. Try lying in bed with no nightie or pyjamas on for an hour each day.
* You could also try applying ice-packs or bags of frozen peas to the area.
* If you feel uncomfortable when you're lying down, try holding a pillow between your legs.
* Begin exercising your pelvic floor muscles (see Chapter 5).

Homoeopathic remedy
* Use Arnica cream or Hypercal ointment around the stitches. Hypericum tincture can also be added to water in a bidet or bowl and used for bathing the area.
* Take Arnica 30C three times a day.
* Bathe the area with a few drops of Calendula tincture in warm water.

Aromatherapy remedy
* Thoroughly mix two drops of lavender oil and one drop of chamomile in a litre of ice-cold water. Sit in the water for a few minutes each day or apply the mixture on a cold compress to the area.
* Add two drops of lavender and two drops of cypress oil to a warm bath. Relax for 10–15 minutes.

CONSTIPATION
This is a fairly common complaint after giving birth. Your vagina and perineum may be so sore that going to the loo is a bit of an ordeal, especially if you have had stitches. Painkilling drugs given during labour can also leave you feeling constipated.

Helping yourself
If you have had an episiotomy, you can support your stitches when you open your bowels by holding a pad against the area. This makes it less painful and less likely that the stitches will give way against the pressure (but this is extremely unlikely).

If you do have constipation, diet is the key for a quick cure. Eat plenty of fibre – found in fresh fruit, vegetables and wholegrains. Try to cut out dairy products or meat and drink plenty of water (at least six glasses a day). Avoid eating a lot of bread and wheat products as gluten can block up your lower digestive tract and aggravate the problem.

POST-NATAL HEALTH

Aromatherapy remedy

Make your own constipation massage remedy: use ten drops of marjoram, ten of rosemary, five of patchouli and five of fennel or juniper. Add these to 50ml of base oil. Massage clockwise over the lower abdomen, concentrating on the left side of the body, following the line of the descending colon.

PILES

These are another post-natal niggle suffered by many women. Piles (or haemorrhoids) are varicose veins of the rectum – caused by increased pressure of the growing uterus during pregnancy on all veins of the pelvis. They may either appear as small round lumps around your back passage or be internal, often being pushed out at the same time as the baby. However, even women who have had Caesarean deliveries can suffer badly from piles. You may find they appear each time you open your bowels, or that they are there all the time.

Helping yourself

Increasing the fibre in your diet to keep your bowels moving may help. You can also try applying compresses soaked in a few drops of witch hazel, bought from your chemist. You can also ask your midwife for a special piles cream. Linseeds taken with water are also an excellent remedy and ease the pain. In extreme cases, a simple surgical operation can be performed to remove both internal and external haemorrhoids and tidy up any loose skin.

Homoeopathic remedy

Use a homoeopathic or herbal piles cream or ointment such as Hamamelis. Or take the remedy Hamamelis 6c.

Aromatherapy remedy

Put two drops of geranium essential oil and one drop of cypress in a bowl of warm water and sit in it for as long as you can. Or, add one drop of geranium and one drop of cypress to about one inch of lubricant jelly or Vaseline and apply twice each day and after bowel movements.

BIRTH AFTERPAINS
After the birth, your contracting uterus may give you some pain. Try to relax during these pains, as tensing up will make it worse.

Homoeopathic remedy
Arnica, taken for bruising, may help these afterpains. If it doesn't help, take Magnesia phosphorica before and after you breastfeed.

INSOMNIA
After the birth, you may be on such a high that you have problems relaxing and getting to sleep.

Aromatherapy remedy
One of the best ways to unwind is to give yourself a luxurious aromatherapy bath before you go to bed. Swish three drops of lavender, mandarin or ylang ylang essential oil into the water and lie back and relax! Or use an aromatherapy burner in your bedroom, adding two to three drops of lavender or ylang ylang oil to the water.

Ask your partner to give you a full massage before you climb into bed. Oils which will help you to unwind include bay, chamomile, lavender, mandarin, marjoram and petitgrain, mixed in a base oil. A couple of drops of lavender essential oil on your pillow also works wonders.

THE BLUES
Feeling weepy for a couple of days after the birth is absolutely normal, but if you feel depressed for any longer, seek professional help (see Chapter 4).

POST-NATAL HEALTH

Aromatherapy remedy
Aromatherapy oils can be a great help if you're feeling down. Make a massage blend using ten drops of bergamot, five drops of grapefruit or lemon, five drops of clary sage or geranium and five of ylang ylang or neroli in 50ml of base oil. Or add any of the above oils to your bath or use in an aromatherapy burner.

If you're feeling especially low, make a special oil using different parts of the orange tree – excellent for helping anxiety and tension. Just add two drops each of neroli, petitgrain and orange oil to your bath and soak until you feel yourself unwind.

FIGHTING FATIGUE
If the birth has left you feeling emotionally and physically washed out, make sure you get some time to yourself to speed up your recovery.

Helping yourself
Ask a relative or your partner to take care of the baby for an hour or two, so you can either get out and treat yourself to a haircut or some pleasurable shopping or simply relax in the bath. Try to stick to a well-balanced diet, and make sure you get out in the fresh air once a day – this helps to blow away those feelings of post-natal lethargy!

Aromatherapy remedy
A morning aromatherapy bath may give you some zest to cope with the rest of the day. Add a couple of drops of geranium or bergamot oil and two to three drops of rosemary to the water. Or use any of the following in a massage oil or bath: lavender, lemon, mandarin, melissa, neroli, rosemary, tangerine and ylang ylang.

SKIN PROBLEMS
Because your hormone levels have changed so dramatically after

the birth, you may find you suffer from a rash or some spots. If you do, try using soothing Calendula cream or echinacea ointment on your spots. Taking 1,000mg evening primrose oil daily can also improve hormonally upset skin.

3

Breastfeeding and Beyond

Breastfeeding is good for mother and baby. Human milk contains essential fatty acids which can help your baby's physical and mental development. Your milk is also good for your baby's brain and blood vessel growth, while protecting him or her from coughs, colds, chest and stomach infections. Breastfed babies have even been found to be marginally more intelligent and have a higher IQ rating possibly due to the presence in breastmilk of unique essential fatty acids needed for brain development. There is also some evidence to show that breastfed babies are less likely to get allergies and are less likely to develop certain diseases in later life. Breastfed babies are also unlikely to become constipated and their stools are soft and not as smelly as those of bottlefed babies.

Feeding a baby with your own milk also means you don't have the hassle of preparing feeds or washing or sterilising bottles. Not only does breastfeeding establish a special bond between you and your baby, it helps your uterus contract after the birth – which means you will get back to your former shape more quickly. It's also free!

But while breastfeeding does give your baby the best possible start in life, it doesn't always come naturally. You may find it painful and have to learn the right way to position your baby on your breast. But don't be discouraged, you may simply need advice on how to breastfeed properly. If you leave hospital soon after the birth, your midwife and health visitor will help you find a comfortable way to feed your baby. And if you feel you need more support, you can get help from a breastfeeding counsellor – either through the La Leche League or the National Childbirth Trust (see Useful Addresses).

Beginning Breastfeeding

Putting your baby to the breast as soon as possible after the birth is the best way to begin feeding. Initially it may be easier for you to feed lying down, especially if you have stitches. Lie on your side with your baby next to you, with his or her mouth in line with your nipple. Support the baby by placing your hand on its shoulders – not behind the head. Then, pulling the baby close to you, offer your breast. Brush your nipple against the baby's lips and then tickle them with the nipple. When your baby opens his or her mouth, pull it up to the breast – and your baby should respond with interest!

You can tell if your baby is correctly positioned if there is more of your areola (the darker coloured area surrounding your nipple) showing above the baby's top lip than below the bottom. Her gums should be working on the areola, not dragging on your nipple, which should be at the back of the mouth. It may help to check where your baby's chin is resting. It should be against your breast – not tilted away from it (as you can't see this, check with your hand). When your baby is in a good position, her lips are pushed right back, instead of in a pout which will mean she is just sucking on your nipple.

If feeding hurts or your baby doesn't seem to be getting enough milk, you may be badly positioned. Stop the feed by putting your little finger in the corner of her mouth, then alter your feeding position and start again.

Breastfeeding tips

- You may like to sit upright supported by cushions or lie down while feeding. But make sure your back is well supported to avoid any backache. Try placing your baby on a pillow, so it is easier for her to reach your breast. Eventually you will find a position which suits both of you.
- Always bring your baby to your breast – not the breast to your baby.
- Don't lean back as your nipple will point upwards, making it hard for your baby to latch on, and don't lean forward over your baby, as the nipples will be pointing downwards, which is also tricky.
- If your breast is heavy, it may help to support it with one hand while you hold the baby with the other hand.

Relaxation

Feeling relaxed is very important for happy breastfeeding – as worry, stress, fatigue and even embarrassment can stop the let-down reflex from working (the pins and needles feeling you get as the milk collects behind the nipple and surrounding area). If relaxation while breastfeeding is a problem, find a quiet place where you can sit and listen to soothing music while feeding. Making a drink such as a cup of tea or glass of milk to have while you breastfeed may also help you to enjoy the experience. You may even like to listen to the radio or watch television while feeding! Rocking chairs are also a wonderful invention for nursing mothers.

You produce less milk when you are run down and tired. So it's vital to eat well and get as much rest as possible. Your baby may want to eat more in the evening, so try to get some rest and eat well during the day.

Your Breastfeeding Diet

Your nutritional needs are very high while breastfeeding – so make sure you're eating well. You particularly need calcium, magnesium, zinc, the B vitamins and folic acid in your diet. Remember that everything you eat will be passed on to your child – so eat plenty of fresh fruit and vegetables to keep you and your baby topped up with many of the essential nutrients. To boost your energy levels try to eat plenty of unrefined carbohydrates and fibre, such as potatoes, wholewheat bread and pasta. Try to avoid junk foods and sweets – these won't help you shed any of the weight you put on while pregnant, and certainly have no nutritional value. To keep your energy levels high, it may help to eat little and often.

You may hear that eating foods such as curries and oranges will affect your milk and give your baby colic. But don't worry – you can probably eat anything while breastfeeding. If you eat something unusual this may affect the baby as he or she isn't used to this type of food. Some babies are also affected by a high-protein diet and it can help to cut out milk or cheese to relieve your baby's colic.

You will probably find you get very thirsty while breastfeeding – so stock up your fridge with plenty of juices, mineral water and milk. Some babies are affected by the caffeine in tea, coffee and cola – it keeps them awake at night – so avoid drinking too much of these. You could try some of the delicious herbal teas now available. Some, such as chamomile, can actually help you to relax.

If you are breastfeeding, smoking is not advisable. Toxins from the cigarette will pass straight through into your breastmilk – not good for a young baby! Smoking has also been linked to increased risk of cot death. You may want the occasional glass of wine or beer to relax but don't overdo it, as alcohol is also passed into your milk and will affect your baby some hours later.

Breastfeeding Problems

SORE OR CRACKED NIPPLES

This is a very common problem in the first couple of weeks of breastfeeding. It may be because your baby is sucking very hard or is in the wrong position at your breast. Try to solve the problem early, because if sore nipples aren't treated quickly, they can develop cracks.

Solutions

* Keep your nipples clean and dry. Change breast pads often and go without a bra occasionally to let fresh air get to your nipples. If it's warm you could try sleeping topless.
* You could try an aromatherapy massage. Using almond oil as a base, add two to three drops of lavender or neroli oil. Roll your nipple between finger and thumb as you massage, immediately after a feed. Make sure you wash your breast thoroughly before the next feed.
* A good homoeopathic cure for sore cracked nipples is to bathe the nipples in Arnica solution (ten drops of tincture to 0.25l of cooled, boiled water).
* For inflamed tender nipples, try using Chamomilla and for cracked nipples which cause smarting, burning pain take Sulphur.
* Gently massage in a Rescue Remedy (one of Bach's well-known Flower Remedies) or chamomile cream after each feed. Specially formulated creams such as Calendula are excellent.
* After each feed, squeeze a little milk from your breast, and smear it over the nipple. This can help protect your nipples.
* Avoid using soap or bubble baths as these can dry your skin.

POST-NATAL HEALTH

ENGORGED BREASTS

New mothers often find that on the third or fourth day after delivery, when their milk comes in, their breasts feel very swollen, hot and uncomfortable. This can also happen later in breastfeeding – particularly if you go without feeding the baby for longer than usual. If your breasts do become engorged you should treat it as quickly as possible, as it could lead to a blocked milk duct which can cause a painful breast infection called mastitis.

Solutions

* Feed as much as possible to reduce the milk build-up in your breasts.
* Take a warm bath with two drops of lavender essential oil and two drops of geranium oil in the water. Soak a flannel in the bath and hold it gently against each breast. This should relieve some of the pressure. Gentle massage with a few drops of fennel essential oil in a light carrier oil (such as peach kernel) is also very effective.
* Draw off some of your milk by expressing it by hand – simply massage the breast over a basin to encourage the milk to flow, or use a breast pump.
* If you are also feeling weepy and sensitive to the cold, many homoeopaths recommend taking Pulsatilla.
* Place ice-cold flannels on your breasts after a feed to reduce the blood supply. To chill the flannel, place ice-cubes inside.
* Take some large chilled green cabbage leaves, soften them with a rolling pin and place them inside your bra to cool down and soothe your breasts. This looks odd – but is highly effective!

BREASTFEEDING AND BEYOND

LUMPY BREASTS
This could be caused by a blocked milk duct and can also lead to mastitis.

Solutions
- * Feed on the tender breast, while smoothing the milk away from where you think the blockage may be.
- * Make sure your bra isn't too tight and nothing is pressing into your breast as you feed, such as your bra or arm.

SORE RED PATCH
If you have a delicate red patch on your breast, you probably have a blocked milk duct. It is important to deal with this quickly or it could develop into mastitis.

Solutions
- * You must get the milk flowing through the duct so warm up your breast by putting a hot flannel over the sore patch and stroke gently from the area down to the nipple.
- * Put the baby on the sore breast as often as you can to encourage your milk flow.

MASTITIS
If you have a hot, tender breast with a red patch you probably have mastitis. You may also have flu-like symptoms, and feel feverish with a temperature and headaches. This infection is usually caused by a blocked milk duct and can be prevented if caught early enough. It is wise to visit your GP or midwife early on to prevent an abscess from developing. You may then be given a course of antibiotics. This does not mean you will have to give up breastfeeding though. Mastitis can be a sign that you are overdoing things or that you are very tired, so try to take it easy for a while.

POST-NATAL HEALTH

Solutions

* The best thing to do is to feed as much as possible from the inflamed breast, as this will help to unblock the milk duct. While this can be very painful, it does eventually help to relieve the problem. So grit your teeth and start each feed off on the infected breast. Try feeding in different positions, as mastitis may also be caused by a bad position – such as being hunched over your baby rather than sitting upright.
* Alternately place hot and cold compresses onto the sore breast every two to four hours.
* While the baby feeds, massage your breast to encourage the duct to unblock.
* Try expressing milk or breastfeeding in the bath to get your milk to flow more readily.
* Place your baby on the breast so that her chin points across from the blocked milk duct. Also try feeding in different positions – sometimes your baby isn't emptying all the ducts as she feeds.
* Do visit your doctor immediately if there is no sign of improvement, as mastitis can lead to a breast abscess. This is caused by pus in the breast and is treated by an incision in the breast which is then drained.
* Do make use of the breastfeeding counsellors available (see Useful Addresses). These women have all had first-hand experience of breastfeeding problems and are generally excellent in a crisis or as a confidante.

TOO MUCH MILK

When your milk first arrives, it may spurt everywhere – or the baby may take too much, become uncomfortable and cry.

Solutions
- Use a nipple shield to decrease the flow of milk.
- Use breast pads inside your bra to absorb any excess drips.
- Express a little milk before you feed, so the baby won't choke if it flows too fast.
- Don't worry – your milk flow will probably even out by the time the baby is eight weeks old.

TOO LITTLE MILK
If your breasts don't provide the constant supply of milk your baby needs, try the following:

Solutions
- Quite simply, try feeding more often. The more your baby feeds, the more milk your breasts will produce.
- Take a short course of the homoeopathic remedy Urtica urens.
- Try using a compress with aromatherapy oils: one drop of fennel, one drop of geranium and one drop of clary sage.
- Drink plenty of fluids. You will need about two pints more each day than you usually have.
- Stop drinking caffeinated drinks as these can reduce your milk supply by overstimulating your nervous system. Drinking fennel tea is also said to increase milk supply.
- Relax! If you're feeling tense your milk supply probably won't be as plentiful as it would if you were calmer. Find a quiet place where you and your baby can focus on the job in hand.
- Increase your food intake and try to get more rest.

Express Yourself

A few weeks after the birth, you may want to leave your baby with a friend or relative so you can have a much needed break. If you're breastfeeding, the best way to provide for your baby in this time is to express some milk from your breasts.

Learning to express can be like learning to breastfeed all over again. Some women find it very easy, while others have real difficulties. One option is to buy a hand or electric breast pump – which can be quicker than expressing milk by hand. If you can't afford an electric pump, you may be able to hire one from your local branch of the National Childbirth Trust or La Leche League (see Useful Addresses). These are excellent machines and well worth the small daily hire charge.

To use the pump, you should sterilise all the equipment and wash your hands. Then splash warm water over your breasts or place warm flannels over them and massage gently. Place the pump over the areola to make an airtight seal and then start pumping! The breast pump works in the same way as your baby's mouth by stimulating your milk ducts to express milk.

Some women find expressing by hand is far easier than using a pump. There are several ways of doing this. First, sterilise a bowl to catch the milk as it comes out. You can try warming your breasts by applying hot flannels and then massaging your breasts for a few minutes. Work your way around the breasts, starting from the top and moving round to the bottom. Do this about ten times to encourage your milk to flow. Sometimes sitting in the bath can help you relax more. Then, stroke your breasts a couple of times with a downwards motion towards the areola. Using your thumbs and forefingers, squeeze your nipple, while pressing backwards at the same time. The milk should now begin to spurt out into the bowl.

Continue to squeeze your breast until it only expresses a few drops, squeezing different parts of the breast so you empty the milk ducts properly. Then move to the other breast and follow the same procedure.

If you're having difficulties expressing more than a couple of drops of breastmilk, try using a pump on one breast while you are feeding on the other, or try just before or after a feed. It may be that you are not completely relaxed about expressing, which can inhibit your milk flow. As with breastfeeding, do it in a place where you feel comfortable and relaxed. Sometimes just sitting in a warm bath with a bowl can work wonders for encouraging your breasts to express milk.

When you have enough milk for a feed, store it in a sterilised, capped bottle in the fridge. But don't keep it for more than twenty-four hours, or it will go off. To keep milk for a few weeks, you can freeze it in special freezer bags, available from good chemists, the National Childbirth Trust and La Leche League. When you need the milk, put it in the fridge until completely defrosted, and don't try to warm it up until it has thawed.

Bottlefeeding

If you can't or simply don't want to breastfeed, bottlefeeding is the answer. Make sure you have at least six bottles and teats, a supply of formula milk and sterilising equipment. Follow the instructions on the formula packet exactly – any extra could harm your baby. You can store ready-prepared bottles in the fridge for up to twenty-four hours.

Sterilise each bottle and teat before use. You can do this by using chemical sterilising tablets or liquid in cold water, or by using a steam steriliser.

TIPS
* As with breastfeeding, you need to be comfortable and relaxed. Hold your baby close to you as you feed her

POST-NATAL HEALTH

and let her have as much milk as she wants. After each feed throw away any leftover milk.

* While you feed, keep the bottle tilted so the teat is full of milk or your baby will take in air.
* If your baby seems unhappy with the bottle, try a different kind of teat. They are available in lots of different shapes and sizes – even nipple-shaped!
* Never leave your baby alone with a bottle in her mouth, or add solids to the milk as this can cause choking.

Combining Breast and Bottle

If you're going back to work, or simply want to be able to leave your baby with someone else from time to time, you can use both breast and formula milk. As teats smell and feel different to your nipples, you should try and get the baby used to the bottle before you actually wish to leave her. Get your partner or a friend to start giving the bottle each day (as your baby will expect milk from the breast from you) at a feed when you intend to be at work or out. You don't have to use powdered milk, you could put expressed breast milk in a bottle. Give your baby about a week to acclimatise to this form of feeding. Then give her another bottle feed, also around the time you intend to be out and about. It could take several weeks for the baby to adjust – but once she is used to a bottle, there is no looking back!

You can then continue to give your baby morning and evening breastfeeds (this usually works best if your baby is over four months old, as your milk supply is then well established). If you find your breasts are full, making your milk squirt out during the day, you can express it during a break at work, and leave it in the fridge to give your baby a feed the following day.

If you wish to continue breastfeeding while you're at work, you can express milk to be given to your baby from a cup or bottle during the day. Or, if you are lucky enough to have an understanding employer, or a crèche at your workplace, you can slip out at the baby's meal times to feed her.

Starting on Solids

Most babies are given their first mouthfuls of solid foods between the ages of four and six months. Before a baby is three months old, her digestive system isn't capable of absorbing foods more complex than babymilk. It is now thought that the later you leave the introduction of solids the better, to avoid the early introduction of certain foods linked to allergy problems and food intolerances. Some doctors suggest leaving it until your baby is at least three-and-a-half months old.

As each baby is different, there is no hard and fast rule about the right age to start eating solids. Let your baby tell you when she is ready to eat solid food. Give it a try when your baby:

* is still hungry after having a good milk feed (eg 225ml or 8fl oz)
* starts to demand more feeds over a long period
* appears more restless than normal, especially at night.

Although you are offering your baby her first few mouthfuls of solids, it is important to remember that the main source of nutrition at this stage is still milk. The amount of breast or formula milk given should not be reduced – the first solids are just an extra to whet your baby's appetite. Start with a small plastic teaspoon of thin porridge made from oat flakes, rice flakes or cornmeal, mixed with a little breast or formula milk. Commercial baby rice is a great starter food. It is very

POST-NATAL HEALTH

convenient and most brands are nutritionally sound. Check that the baby rice you use is completely salt and sugar free.

How to Wean

Give your baby the new food in the middle or at the end of a milk feed, as she will be more receptive to the idea once her initial hunger pangs have been satisfied. For the first two weeks, just give the solids to your baby once a day, and gradually build it up until you are giving solids at three feeds a day.

Offer your baby some new flavours after a couple of weeks, but leave a few days between each new flavour as taste is a new experience to a baby. This will also give you the chance to look out for any allergic reaction to food, such as diarrhoea or skin rashes.

Try offering a little vegetable or fruit purée (without any salt or sugar) on the tip of a clean teaspoon. You could try potato, carrot, parsnip, plantain, broccoli, spinach, pear, apple or banana. If your baby refuses a food, don't force it – just try again a couple of weeks later, when she may be more enthusiastic.

WEANING TIPS
* Babies are often more receptive to solids when they are in the feeding position.
* Try to relax while weaning. If you make a big issue out of food, weaning will become a harder task for both of you.
* Be prepared for a mess – have plenty of wipes, a bib and a muslin cloth at hand.
* To save time, it's easier to make a whole batch of purée and freeze it in small quantities. If your baby is very young, try using a plastic ice-cube tray to freeze small meal-sized portions. For the older baby, plastic pots or

yoghurt cartons (well washed) with a foil cover are ideal. Remember not to keep anything for too long in the freezer; label and date without fail, so you know exactly what everything is.

* Buy a couple of the shallow plastic baby teaspoons to make weaning easier.
* You won't need any extra kitchen equipment to make baby food. All the foods mentioned above can be made with a few pots and pans, a fork, grater and a sieve. But you may find a blender or food processor is very useful.

What to avoid

Don't give your baby any salt, sugar or fatty foods. And avoid all of the following:

* milk apart from breast or formula milk
* all other dairy products including cheese
* eggs
* wheat-based foods such as wheat cereals and pasta
* citrus fruits
* summer fruits such as strawberries and raspberries.

All these can produce an allergic reaction, so are better left until the baby is a few months older.

Also avoid tomatoes, spices, chillies and nuts. Tomatoes can be introduced at six months and spices and chillies at nine months. Nuts are generally not suitable for babies and young children as they can cause choking, although finely ground nuts can be introduced at nine months.

Weaning recipes (four to six months)

All the purées in this section should be made to a smooth consistency and slightly on the runny side. There are plenty of other fruit and vegetables you can try, but these are good first-time suggestions.

Cereals

Baby rice: This is widely available and should be made up according to the instructions on the packet. Only use rice with no added sugar or salt.

Brown, wholegrain rice: Wash the rice with cold water (the easiest way is to use a sieve under the tap). Simmer in water for about 40 minutes until the grains are tender. Purée using a little baby milk or water to obtain the desired consistency.

Vegetables

Carrot/broccoli/cauliflower: Peel and slice the carrot, or separate the broccoli or cauliflower into small florets. Simmer in water for about 10 minutes. Purée with a blender or through a sieve, adding a little of the cooking water to obtain a smooth texture.

Courgette: Wash, trim the ends and slice. Simmer for about 5 minutes until tender. (Courgettes also steam very well but need slightly longer – 8–12 minutes.) Purée.

Potato/sweet potato/parsnip/turnip/swede: Peel and dice the vegetable. Simmer in water until tender (about 20 minutes). Mash well with a fork, using some of the cooking water to obtain the right consistency.

Fruit

Apple/pear: Peel and core the fruit (use an eating apple as it will need no added sugar). Chop into pieces, place in a pan and cover with water. Simmer gently until soft (5–10 minutes). Purée.

Banana: Mash 1/4–1/2 of a ripe banana thoroughly with a fork. It may need a little cooled, boiled water or breast or formula milk to obtain a smooth purée. (Banana does not freeze well.)

Peach/apricot/nectarine: Submerge the fruit briefly in boiling water and then in cold water to make peeling easier. Peel the fruit, remove the stone and chop the flesh. Steam for 3–5 minutes and then purée.

Cream of ...
Another variation of the basic purée which works well is to make a creamy variety. Simply mix the purée with some baby rice or some breast or formula milk. Your baby may prefer the creamier taste.

For more information, recipes and weaning tables, read my *Quick Guide to Baby and Toddler Foods*.

4

The Baby Blues

Having a baby can be a terrific shock to a woman – so it is not surprising that some women feel low after giving birth. This feeling can range from being a little down and weepy for a couple of days after the birth, to a more serious, seemingly unshakeable depression, which can appear at any time in the first year of your baby's life.

Post-natal Depression

There are three kinds of post-natal depression. The first, and the most common, is the 'baby blues' which affects about 50–80 percent of women. The baby blues is the weepiness, depression and mild irritation many women feel from three to five days after giving birth. The cause of this is thought to be physical so if you do feel down, don't blame yourself. After giving birth the levels of the two main pregnancy hormones – progesterone and oestrogen – drop dramatically. By the third day after the birth these have reached very low levels. These two hormones were responsible for a feeling of wellbeing, which you may have felt during pregnancy. So don't feel surprised if, around day three after your baby's birth, you feel low and start to cry for no apparent reason.

But there are other reasons behind the blues. If your baby has jaundice or another minor problem, you may feel down during the first week. Or, when you get home from the hospital, you may suddenly feel as if you are unable to cope, without the

POST-NATAL HEALTH

back-up of the midwives. This is often the case with your first baby. You may also have had a difficult and exhausting birth which may make you feel tired and uncomfortable for several weeks afterwards. If your baby is very demanding and needs to feed a lot during the night, you may also feel low – lack of sleep after the birth doesn't exactly help to cheer you up!

If you are affected, try to get lots of sleep, give yourself some hot baths with your favourite essential oils and, above all, talk to someone close to you about the way you are feeling. You should be over the baby blues in a couple of days.

The second type of post-natal depression can happen much later – in fact, any time up to a year after your baby is born. This may not begin until several weeks after the birth of the baby and develops more gradually than the baby blues. The symptoms of this more serious problem include depression, lack of energy, a feeling of futility, fatigue, hair loss, insomnia and a loss of interest in sex. All of these symptoms can be mild to moderate.

If you develop post-natal depression you may feel depressed and quite hopeless soon after your baby is born. You may find yourself in tears for no particular reason and may even feel you have been rejected by your partner, family and friends, and sometimes even by the new baby. You may also feel permanently exhausted and unable to cope with everyday chores such as the housework. You may also feel anxious about a variety of things, which wouldn't usually bother you. You might worry about your health and feel pains which your doctor can't diagnose. Other typical symptoms of post-natal depression are a general feeling of illness or permanent tiredness and being too worried even to leave the house. Everyday situations may worry you if you're suffering from post-natal depression. You find it hard to relax and should really avoid situations which cause you concern.

A mother suffering from post-natal depression may have obsessional thoughts about a person, situation or a particular activity. She may become very frightened and worry that she might harm a member of her family or even the baby. She will probably find it difficult to concentrate on books, television or even a conversation. She may also have problems sleeping, with fitful light sleep or waking up with nightmares. Her sex life may also suffer as she completely loses interest in lovemaking.

Puerperal psychosis is the name of the most severe form of post-natal depression, but thankfully it is quite rare. It usually occurs in the first three months after childbirth. Sufferers find it impossible to carry on normally and often suffer manic or depressive symptoms. Treatment of puerperal psychosis is exactly the same as that of any other manic illness – professional advice, reassurance, treatment with appropriate drugs and perhaps a stay in hospital.

Avoiding the Blues

Post-natal depression doesn't have to be inevitable – there are certain ways of beating the blues before they get to you! Try the following suggestions if you're feeling at all down:

* If you are feeling stressed or tired, try to talk about the way you feel to a partner or a good friend – just to release some of your tension. Think about yourself for a change, and how you're feeling, rather than always focusing on the baby or your partner.
* Remember – there's no such thing as the perfect mother and, if your baby is crying all the time, it isn't your fault, it's just the way she is feeling at that moment in time. Contact a support group such as Cry-SIS, the National Childbirth Trust or Meet-a-Mum (see Useful Addresses), which will put you in touch with other parents who have suffered the same problems.

POST-NATAL HEALTH

* Constantly missing a good night's sleep can lead to depression – continually broken sleep cycles have been used as a form of torture! If you are desperate for an unbroken night's sleep, get your partner or a close relative to take over for a night with a bottle of formula milk, or express some milk during the day, and leave it in the fridge for the night feed.
* Take a break from your baby once in a while – if you're constantly there for her, you may begin to feel trapped and resentful. Ask a friend or relative to look after her for a couple of hours and go and do something you enjoy – such as an aerobics class or a trip to the cinema.
* Make sure you eat a well-balanced diet with plenty of fresh fruit and vegetables. A multivitamin supplement is worth taking for a while, as is an iron supplement. Give up caffeinated drinks such as tea, coffee and fizzy drinks as they may make you irritable and anxious, increasing the risk of post-natal depression. Try to eat foods rich in potassium such as bananas, tomatoes and oranges, as you may experience potassium loss after the birth.
* Try to exercise once or twice a week as this will stimulate your endorphins – your body's natural painkillers and mood enhancers. It will also get you out of the house and give you a valuable break from your baby. Many sports centres now have a crèche where you can leave your baby from an early age (some take babies from six weeks old).

Coping with Post-natal Depression

If you have some of the symptoms of post-natal depression and they have lasted longer than a few days, see your doctor or health visitor as soon as possible. Being able to talk to someone sympathetic may help to see you through this difficult time.

If you decide to visit your doctor, tell him or her about *all* your symptoms as this will help to diagnose exactly what you are suffering from. If the doctor thinks your depression is caused by your hormones, and you are on the contraceptive pill, then a change of pill may be suggested (or a new form of contraception such as the cap). If your depression is particularly bad your doctor may prescribe treatment in the form of tranquillisers or antidepressants. Do think about whether you really want this kind of treatment and discuss it fully with your doctor.

Find out which kind of drug you have been prescribed (both have advantages and disadvantages). Mild doses of a moderate tranquilliser such as diazepam can reduce post-natal depression, but all tranquillisers may mask calmer intervals experienced during depression. Tranquillisers can relieve feelings of anxiety quite quickly, but are actually suppressing these feelings as they are treating the symptoms, not the cause. These drugs should really only be taken for a short period of time, as they can be physically and psychologically addictive after two or three months. Tranquillisers can also be passed into your breastmilk and make your baby sleepy – making breastfeeding quite hard going and possibly even dangerous.

Coming off tranquillisers should be done under the supervision of a doctor or psychiatrist, in case you suffer any withdrawal symptoms. These can range from a worsening of the original anxiety to insomnia and new symptoms such as palpitations, nausea and loss of appetite.

Your doctor is more likely to prescribe antidepressant drugs if you have severe post-natal depression. The most common of these are the tricyclic antidepressants – lofetramine (brand name Gamanil), dothiepin (brand name Prothiaden) and trimipramine (brand name Surmantil). You cannot become addicted to these drugs, but you may find if you are taking the tricyclic type that your mouth becomes dry and you feel slightly drowsy. These symptoms will wear off as you continue to take the drug. Tricyclics take up to three weeks to reach their full effect.

More powerful antidepressant drugs are called monoamine oxidase inhibitors (MAOI), and you may be given these if the tricyclic types do not work. But MAOIs can have life-threatening side-effects if you eat foods which contain tyramine, such as ripe cheese, yeast, meat extracts and alcohol. These drugs do work quickly, taking ten days to two weeks to have a curative effect. Like tranquillisers, antidepressants are passed into your breastmilk, but don't appear to have any side-effects on the baby.

Psychotherapy

If you are very depressed, you may want to discuss your problems with a psychotherapist. Take enormous care when choosing a therapist, as it's vital that this person is the right one for you. Ask if you can have an initial meeting with the therapist, to ensure you feel comfortable with him or her. If your instincts tell you this is the wrong person to discuss your feelings with, then look for someone else. You may feel happier seeing a female therapist who has also had children and can relate directly to your experience.

Natural Tranquillisers

If you don't want to take an orthodox drug treatment for postnatal depression, you could try a natural tranquilliser. Some vitamin and mineral supplements can have a calming effect, although they take more time to work than drug treatment:

THE BABY BLUES

- **Vitamin B1** or thiamine can help reduce anxiety. Take 50–100mg each day, together with a calcium supplement.
- **Vitamin B3** is also a useful natural tranquilliser. Take 25–100mg each day.
- **Vitamin B6** may act as a tranquilliser and can help to fight depression. Take 25–100mg each day.
- **Vitamin C** can help to fight stress, particularly if you smoke (this habit reduces blood oxygen level, which then increases your production of lactic acid and increases tension and fatigue). Take 100–500mg each day.
- **Magnesium** is the essential mineral for the effective functioning of the central nervous system. Take a dosage of 200–400mg each day.
- **Zinc** is known for its beneficial effect on the immune system, yet can also have a calming effect on your central nervous system. Take 10–75mg daily.

To simplify your supplement intake, take a **B-complex** vitamin pill (containing B1, B2, B3, B6 and B12) with every meal; a good **iron** supplement and a **calcium** supplement each day.

Self Help

Try these alternative ways to beat post-natal depression:

Do

- Make sure your diet has plenty of raw fruits and vegetables, and eat protein frequently. Drink plenty of fluids and try to have raw vegetable and fruit juice during the day. Try to eat little and often.
- Cut out caffeine as it may be making you feel irritable

POST-NATAL HEALTH

and anxious. Try drinking herbal teas such as chamomile, raspberry and peppermint instead.

* Take some form of exercise every day, even if you just walk to the shops with baby and pushchair. Just getting out of your home and seeing some other people can help you feel better.
* Make sure you take a break from the baby occasionally. This may only be for a couple of hours a week – you can go for a swim or a walk on your own or simply just have a lovely hot bath, in peace. Find a babysitter so you and your partner can have a night out together when you need some time alone.
* Get as much rest as possible, especially if your baby wakes often during the night. Try to have a nap or lie on the sofa at least once a day.
* Try using an alternative therapy such as aromatherapy to lift your depression. Choose a couple of essential oils you really like and put a few drops in a hot bath, then soak for a long time. Oils which can help relieve depression include bay, bergamot, clary sage, geranium, jasmine, neroli, petitgrain, rose, sage, sandalwood, tangerine and ylang ylang. Or make up a massage oil using some of these oils and ask your partner or a friend to give you a really soothing massage. Alternatively, make your own inhalation – mix together twenty drops of clary sage and ten drops of rose otto and store the mixture in a dark glass bottle. Each morning and evening, sprinkle a few drops on a tissue and inhale. You can try the same mix in a vaporiser, for an uplifting effect.
* Try to keep in touch with at least one other mother and baby so you can discuss how each of you feels about parenthood. It may help if you know someone else who has found being a mother quite difficult and tiring, too. Not many women find motherhood easy!

THE BABY BLUES

- ✱ Write down how you're feeling. You might want to describe the birth and how you felt afterwards. Or, if you're finding it hard to cope now – how and why. Expressing your emotions in this way can often help you to understand yourself better.
- ✱ Talk about it. Find another mother who has been through the same thing, or a sympathetic close friend or relative you can open up to. If there is no one you can talk to, visit your health visitor or doctor.

Don't

- ✱ Neglect yourself. Once a week, spoil yourself a little – whether it's with a new haircut, a magazine or a trip to the cinema.
- ✱ Wait until you are at your wits' end before you ask for help. The sooner you can sort out the way you feel, the better.
- ✱ Go on a diet or neglect regular meals. Low blood sugar will make you feel worse if you're feeling low already.
- ✱ Make yourself do things you really don't feel like doing or which tend to upset you. Treat yourself gently.
- ✱ Blame yourself for the way you feel or for your baby's crying – especially if she cries constantly. You will eventually return to normal, and all babies cry, although some more than others!

5

Getting Back Into Shape

This is one of the priorities for every new mother! When you've had your baby, you will obviously feel much lighter, but look down and you will see a flabby tummy. You may also have put on weight on the rest of your body during pregnancy. If you feel relatively well after the birth, the best tip for getting your body back into shape is to start exercising as soon as possible with some gentle stretching exercises.

If you exercise gently each day, gradually building up the type and amount of exercise, you should be able to regain your pre-pregnant figure in about three months. But do take it slowly at first as your ligaments are still soft. And stop as soon as you feel tired, or if you feel you are straining any muscles.

If you've had a Caesarean you shouldn't start doing any of these exercises (apart from the pelvic floor exercise) for at least a few weeks after the birth. Your doctor or midwife will tell you when you're ready to start.

Week One

Why not start toning yourself up before you've even got out of bed? During late pregnancy the muscles running down the middle of your abdomen (recti muscles) may have separated into two halves. So it's important not to push yourself too hard in the early days and to begin with some very gentle movements. From the day after you've given birth you can do these very simple exercises:

POST-NATAL HEALTH

* As you breathe out, gently pull in your abdominal muscles and hold for a few seconds. Then relax slowly. You can do this as often as you like – it will prepare you for the more vigorous abdominal exercises later.
* To improve your circulation while you're still recovering from the birth, try some foot pedalling. Simply bend your feet up and down from your ankles. Then try circling your feet round one way and the other. You can do this several times a day, while you're still lying down.
* Lie with your legs straight, then press your knees hard down onto the bed. Relax. Then clench and relax your buttocks. Bend and stretch each knee to relax your legs.

A few days after the birth you can try this more energetic exercise for your stomach muscles:

* Lie on your back with head and shoulders resting on a couple of pillows. Bend your legs and keep them slightly apart. Then cross your arms over your stomach. Slowly lift your head and shoulders and, as you do, press gently on each side of your tummy with your hands, as if you are pulling both sides together. Hold for a few seconds, breathe in and then relax. Try to repeat several times.

You can combine this exercise with a pelvic rock:

* Lying in the same position as for the previous exercise, breathe out, and push the floor or the bed with your feet. Let your pelvis roll in, so your lower back flattens. Gently push the floor or bed with your feet, so your pelvis rolls and lets your lower back arch. If you unfold your arms and let them lie on the floor or bed while

you do this, you can do this exercise with your baby lying on your stomach!

PELVIC FLOOR EXERCISES

One of the most important exercises you can do immediately after giving birth is to begin to firm up your pelvic floor muscles. The pelvic floor is a very important group of muscles, yet many women know very little about them – this is a shame as they are important not just for pregnancy and birth, but for your whole life! These muscles lie at the bottom of the pelvis, supporting the womb, bladder and bowels, rather like a hammock. The pelvic floor is shaped rather like a figure of eight – a large loop controls the urethra and vagina and a smaller ring at the back controls the anal sphincter. These two rings overlap in the centre, the perineum.

If your pelvic floor weakens, you can suffer from a minor leak of urine each time you cough, laugh, sneeze or even run for the bus. During birth these muscles are particularly important, as the pelvic floor has to relax and stretch to allow the baby to pass through the vaginal opening.

After the birth, the pelvic floor may weaken, so it's important to begin to firm up these muscles as soon as possible. You can tell if your pelvic floor is weak if you suffer from some of these symptoms: low backache; being incontinent if you laugh, sneeze, cough or exercise vigorously; having to pass water frequently, even if there is hardly anything there; piles; pain when you empty your bowels and/or bowel incontinence.

To find out where your pelvic floor actually is, try stopping yourself next time you are urinating. Just stop mid-stream and hold briefly, then empty your bladder. It's the muscles you use to stop the flow that you should be using in pelvic floor exercises. Don't try this experiment more than about once a week, or you may begin not to empty your bladder properly – and avoid it if you have a bladder infection such as cystitis.

POST-NATAL HEALTH

When you've established where these muscles are, try doing this simple exercise every day. Choose a position you feel comfortable in – it may be lying on your back with your knees up, or simply sitting on a chair. Now, slowly pull yourself in and tighten up from around the back passage through to the middle and then the front. Try to hold for four to five counts and then let go. Aim to do five to ten at first and then gradually build up until you are doing about fifty each day.

When you first begin pelvic floor exercises, you may have to concentrate quite hard. But eventually it will become very easy and you'll be able to do it more than once a day. You can exercise your pelvic floor when you are changing the baby's nappy, sitting at traffic lights or waiting to be served in a shop – in fact, anywhere, any time!

If you have had stitches, exercising your pelvic floor will help them to heal more quickly. If sitting up is uncomfortable, try lying on your front to relieve any pressure on the area. Try putting a couple of pillows under your hips – this may help your pelvic organs return to their former position – and put another pillow under your head. Don't push yourself up with your elbows as this puts strain on your back. Try practising your pelvic floor exercises in this position.

Week Two

Now you can start to do slightly more demanding exercises, gradually building up the number you do each day.

TONING YOUR STOMACH MUSCLES

Curling down
Sit on the floor with your legs bent and arms folded. Breathe out and slowly lean back until you feel your stomach muscles

tighten up. Hold in this position for as long as you can. Then, breathing in, slowly sit up straight.

Try the same exercise with your baby! Keeping your legs close together, let your baby lie against your thighs. Slowly lean back, while lengthening your legs at the same time. When you feel your abdominal muscles tighten, pull yourself back up, moving as close to your knees as possible.

Curling up
Lie on the floor with legs bent and arms at your sides. Tighten your abdominal muscles. Then, bringing your chin to your chest, curl up as far as you can, gradually stretching your hands to your feet. Slowly lower yourself back to the floor.

Side bends
Lie on the floor with your legs bent, arms by your sides. Tighten your abdominal muscles and slowly raise your head and shoulders. As you do this, slide your right hand to touch your right foot and bend sideways. Then straighten up and repeat on your left-hand side.

Leg limber
You can do this exercise with your baby lying on your tummy or chest. Lie on your back with your knees bent. Place one hand in the small of your back and then push against the floor with your feet, squeezing your hand. Then, keeping the pressure on your hand, slide your feet forward, lengthening your legs. See how far you can move your legs. As they push down, your stomach muscles begin to work. Press on your hand more firmly with your back and let your toes come up so your leg muscles don't tense up. If you feel the small of your back coming up off the floor, don't push your legs down any further. Bring each foot back to the starting position separately and start again.

POST-NATAL HEALTH

Begin with five of the above exercises each day, and gradually increase to twenty.

EXERCISING WITH BABY

You may like to do these fun movements with your baby, which will also help to tone you up!

Arm lift

A great exercise for mother and baby. Lie on the floor with your knees bent. Place your baby on your chest and hold her under her arms. Then gently lift her into the air, over your face. You should feel your lower back pressing into the floor as you do this. Hold her in this position for as long as it feels comfortable and then lower her back down to your chest.

Pelvic rocking

This is good for your back and bottom muscles and your baby will love it, too! Lie on your back with your knees bent. Hold your baby on your chest. Then, slowly lift your back and bottom off the floor, so there is a horizontal line running from feet to shoulders. Hold yourself like this for a few seconds. Gently sway from side to side, letting your pelvis rock. Then return to your first position.

Moving On

After a few weeks of doing the above exercises, you should begin to get more toned. You can then think about starting a more energetic exercise routine – perhaps even going to a gentle aerobics class or swimming a few lengths at your local pool. This will not only help you return to your former fitness, but will give you more energy and vitality. It may also give you a short break from your baby if you leave her with a friend or in a crèche. If

GETTING BACK INTO SHAPE

you can't find a minder, simply going for a walk with your baby every day in the fresh air will help you back to fitness.

Relaxation

Looking after a small baby is great fun, but also very tiring. You may feel you have no time left to yourself and find it hard to relax when you do have a moment's peace. This is why finding an effective form of relaxation is vital – whether with a hot bath or simply a few minutes' quiet contemplation. Or you could try these simple exercises, based on yoga postures. The best time to do them is when your baby is asleep or being looked after by someone else, so you will relax properly.

Breathing exercise
It might sound odd, but learning to breathe properly can really help you to relax. Practising breathing exercises every day will also help you cope with the busy schedule of being a new mother. You may find you get less tense or uptight as a result of doing these exercises.

To do breathing exercises you need to find a quiet room, which isn't too stuffy or too cold. If it's warm outside you might like to try this in the park or your garden. Sit on the floor with your legs folded or crossed or, if it's more comfortable, stretch them out in front of you or place a pillow against your back.

Close your eyes and try and focus on yourself, letting all other thoughts and worries drift away. Think about your breathing. As you breathe out, let your body relax. Let your chin drop down to your chest, relax your shoulders, stomach and pelvic floor. Put your hands on your tummy and concentrate on your breathing. Then begin to breathe out through your mouth and in through your nose. As you exhale, contract your abdominal muscles sharply, raising your diaphragm and forcing air

POST-NATAL HEALTH

from your lungs. When you inhale, relax the muscles and let your lungs fill up with air. Make the exhalation quite brief, the inhalation longer. Continue to breathe in this way for several minutes, after which you can place your hands palm upwards on your knees. Then, just focus on your breathing and sit calmly for a while.

This exercise can be done anywhere at any time – just as long as you have some peace and quiet and space to yourself.

Meditation

If you find the breathing useful, you may like to try a little simple meditation. Sit in a comfortable position – perhaps cross-legged or in the lotus position (see page 69). Before you begin, try to tell your mind to calm down and to forget all current worries. Start with the breathing exercise for several minutes, letting your mind wander. Establish a rhythmic breathing pattern – inhaling then exhaling for about three seconds. Try to bring your mind to rest – perhaps place a candle or other object in front of you to focus on. Then hold your concentration on this object, continuing to breathe slowly. If you can detach yourself from your everyday thoughts and concentrate on your mind, you will have reached a meditative state. It may take a few times to actually achieve this but, once you have, you will probably want to do it every day.

GETTING BACK INTO SHAPE

Neck and shoulder release

You may have accumulated tension in your neck and shoulders – this can result in stiffness, bad posture and even headaches.

Sit on the floor with your legs crossed and back straight, looking straight ahead. Slowly drop your head back and then bring it forwards onto your chest. Then, with your head upright, turn it round to the right and then back round to the left. Then, drop your head forwards and roll it all the way around. Repeat this in the opposite direction. Raise your right shoulder and drop it down. Repeat this with your left shoulder. Then raise both shoulders at once and drop them down. Repeat each of these movements five times.

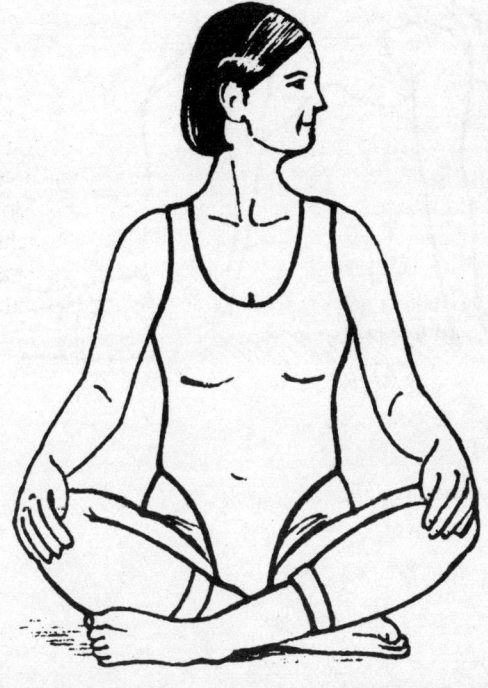

POST-NATAL HEALTH

The cat
Get down onto all fours. Place your hands shoulder distance apart and your knees slightly apart. Then, breathing out, arch your back up, slowly. At the same time lower your neck. Breathing in, flatten your back and raise your head. Repeat five times.

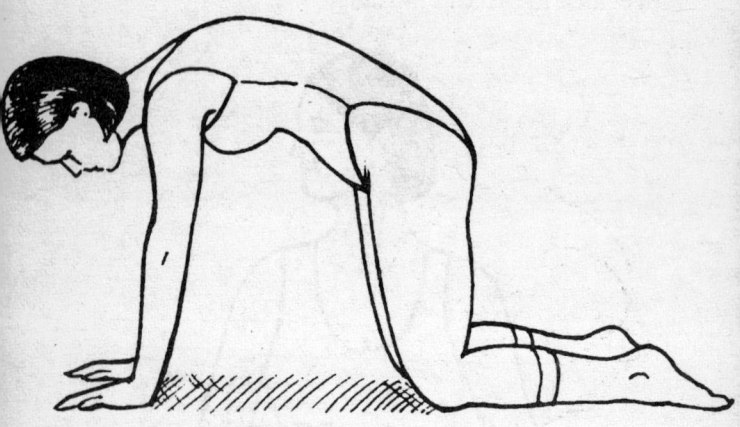

GETTING BACK INTO SHAPE

The frog

Kneel on the floor, separating your knees with your feet together. Then sit back on your heels. Breathe in and then breathe out slowly, pushing your hands forward on the floor, with your head down. Try to stretch your spine as far as you can. Move your fingers further across the floor and gradually let your head rest between your arms. Feel that stretch! Then, fold your arms and rest your head on them. Do your pelvic floor exercise ten times in this position (see page 64).

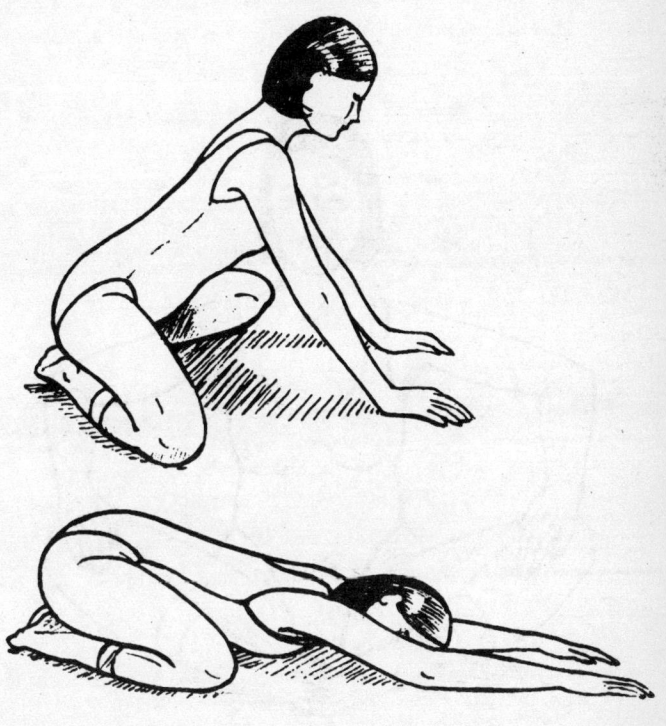

POST-NATAL HEALTH

Sit and stretch

Sit upright on the floor, with your spine held up and the back of your neck straight. Then stretch your legs wide apart. Place your hands on your knees and gently breathe in and out as you feel the stretch. Then, bring the soles of your feet together and gently let your knees drop towards the floor. (Don't worry if they won't drop – this will take time.) Then take some more slow, even breaths.

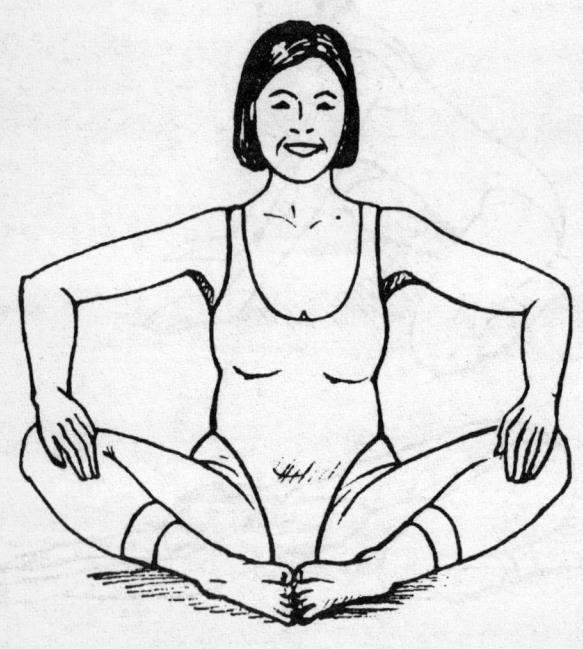

GETTING BACK INTO SHAPE

The lotus

This position encourages you to sit upright and breathe deeply – essential for proper relaxation. It also encourages flexibility in ankles, knees and hips, as well as being good for the nerves in your legs.

Sit on the floor with your legs bent – soles of the feet together. For the simple lotus, just press your knees forward with your hands. To sit in the lotus position, splay your legs in front of you in a V-shape. Then, bend one knee and bring the foot in towards you, placing it as high as you can on your thigh. Now, bring the other foot in and place on the opposite thigh. Sit in this position for a few minutes, breathing in and out slowly (as for the breathing exercise on page 67). You may like to close your eyes and drift off.

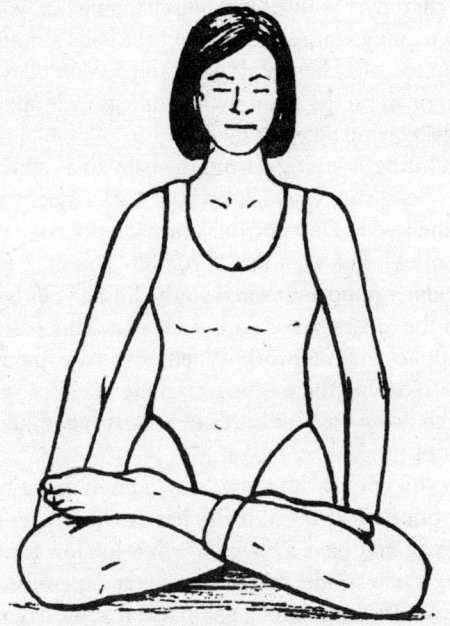

POST-NATAL HEALTH

Your Back

For several months after the birth, you should try to take great care of your back, particularly when lifting and bending. This is because your ligaments are still very soft and any sudden, jerky movements could seriously strain your back. It is particularly important that you take good care of your back if you have had an epidural – as you are more likely to suffer from backache. All the abdominal exercises above will help to strengthen your back, and care taken while lifting and carrying will also help avoid backache. Try following these tips to avoid getting a bad back:

* The way you hold yourself while doing housework or changing nappies can affect your back. If you have to bend right over your baby while changing her, you aren't helping yourself. Either put the baby's changing mat on top of a chest of drawers so you don't have to strain, or sit on the floor, with your legs wide apart and your baby lying between them.
* When lifting anything – from the baby to a carrycot – always bend your knees, keep your back straight and hold the weight close to your body. Try to make your thigh muscles do the work as you lift. This is particularly important when you're lifting your baby out of the Moses basket, cot or car seat. This position also applies to housework. Whether you are making beds, unloading the washing machine or cleaning the bath, go down on bent knees to a squatting or kneeling position.
* When you're out with the baby in a pram or pushchair, keep your back straight. If you have to bend over to push, you may have a buggy which is too low for you. Buying a new model might sound very expensive, but it will save you the pain of a bad back! If you carry your

GETTING BACK INTO SHAPE

baby in a sling, make sure it doesn't put too much pressure on any one part of your back – the weight should be evenly distributed.

* If you find your sink unit is too low and you have to bend over to do the washing up, place a bowl upside-down in the sink with another bowl on top. Or try sitting on a stool with your knees tucked into the cupboard below. (Also, sit on a stool for brushing your teeth, etc. in the bathroom.)
* Feeding your baby should be done in a comfortable place, with a good support for your back. If you find yourself hunching over, put a cushion on your lap to raise the baby closer to your breasts. If you feed your baby in bed, make sure you have enough pillows behind your back to support it from the bottom to the top of your spine.
* If you drive a lot, ensure your back is well supported by adjusting the seat until it feels right.

6

Natural Baby Care

Learning about your baby during the first few weeks is a truly magical and exciting experience. You will see her change each week as you gradually get to know one another. While your baby is beginning to get to know you, she is also discovering about the world.

Bonding with your baby may not happen overnight. You may take a few weeks to get to know her, and she is also learning all about you! That's why close physical contact with your newborn is so important. Touching your baby will establish a loving bond between the pair of you and is an excellent way to communicate. Bathing your baby regularly or gentle massage are great ways of establishing a close relationship.

Giving Your Baby a Massage

Follow these simple tips if you're going to massage your baby:

- ✱ Find a warm room, without too many distractions.
- ✱ Have your baby's changing mat, a clean nappy and a towel handy.
- ✱ Only start the massage if your baby is happy – if she is hungry or tired, it will be a waste of time. Giving a massage after your baby's bath is a good time.
- ✱ Equally, make sure you aren't tired or in a hurry. Your baby will pick up on this and the massage won't be as enjoyable.

POST-NATAL HEALTH

- ✱ Talk only to your baby – chatting to someone else will simply distract her from the massage.
- ✱ Talk or sing to your baby throughout the massage to make it an enjoyable experience for her.
- ✱ Make sure your nails are short and you aren't wearing jewellery, which could scratch your baby.
- ✱ If your baby isn't enjoying the massage, stop immediately. You could try again in a few days. It should be a fun time for both of you.

BABY MASSAGE OIL

Use a vegetable oil as a carrier for the essential oils, rather than baby oil, as the former is more easily absorbed by your baby's skin. For a simple massage oil, simply add one drop of lavender oil to 100ml (5tbsp) of almond oil. Or try adding two drops of Roman chamomile, rose or neroli or lavender oil to 100ml of almond oil, or to 80ml of almond oil and 20ml of jojoba oil.

Caution: Never use any more essential oils than the amounts recommended above. Babies and small children should only ever have tiny amounts. Never use neat essential oils on your baby's skin.

THE BABY MASSAGE

To begin the massage, sit on the floor with your legs wide apart. Place a large towel on your lap and put the baby on top, lying on her back. You can do any part of this massage, or the entire thing. Try not to massage for more than ten minutes at a time as your baby may get either bored or overstimulated. Follow this procedure:

- ✱ **Front.** This may be all your baby wants massaged at first. Using the palms of your hands, massage up the sides of her body, and then up to his or her chest.

Gently massage your baby's tummy from one side and then back to the other again.

* **Arms.** Circle your fingers around the shoulders and then glide your hands gently down to the wrists and back up to the shoulders. Repeat three times.
* **Legs.** Use both your hands to massage a small amount of oil from her ankles up to the tops of her legs. Then gently move your hands back down to her feet, without putting any pressure on her legs. Repeat three times. If you want to spend more time on her legs, massage each one separately – begin with the calf and foot and then massage the thigh.
* **Feet.** Take each foot with your hand. Using your thumbs, massage each sole with circular movements, swapping directions halfway through. Try this several times. This massage can be very calming for a baby and may be useful to soothe her when crying.
* **Back.** Turn your baby over onto her tummy, so she's lying across your thighs. Place one hand on her bottom and, with the other, massage from the top of her back to her bottom. Then massage the back of her legs from ankles to bottom. You can try this in one movement – holding the baby by her ankles, massage from her shoulders right down to her calves.

Caution: Remember not to massage your baby's hands as the oil could be passed into her mouth. It's probably better to avoid massaging the face, as oil could also get into her eyes or mouth.

Baby Skin Care

Your baby's soft skin is very delicate and needs to be treated with great care. So avoid using standard infant bubble baths

POST-NATAL HEALTH

which are based on detergent and choose liquid emollient baths such as Oilatum or Wash E45, or try one of the baby hypo-allergenic ranges now available. If your baby is over a month old, give her skin a chance to breathe each day by giving an air bath. Just take off clothes and nappy in a warm room and let your baby kick about on a changing mat for half an hour. Most babies love the opportunity to feel the air on their skin.

AVOIDING NAPPY RASH

If the area around your baby's genitals becomes spotty, red and sore, then she probably has nappy rash. This usually happens when a nappy has been left on for too long. If you're using fabric nappies, this could also be an allergy to soap powder and fabric conditioner.

To avoid this problem, change your baby's nappy often and clean and dry her bottom thoroughly at each change. Whenever you can, let your baby lie around without a nappy to expose her to the air. If you are using terry nappies, don't use a biological powder or fabric conditioner to clean them as these can encourage an allergy.

If your baby does develop nappy rash:

* Wash your baby's genitals thoroughly with lukewarm water – without using soap. Make sure you clean all the little creases properly.
* Leave your baby without a nappy for as long as possible. You could try leaving her for a few hours in the cot on a layer of towels placed over a plastic sheet.
* Try using a different type of disposable nappy, perhaps a more absorbent brand. If you're using terry nappies, change the soap powder.
* You can buy nappy rash creams at the chemist. Sudocrem is one of the most effective. Apply after you have cleaned her skin.

NATURAL BABY CARE

* Try using Calendula or Symphytum ointment after each change of nappy.

CRADLE CAP

This is when your baby's head is covered in either white scaly patches or brown crusty patches. It is caused by the glands in your baby's hair follicles overproducing oil.

* Don't pick off the dry patches, but gently smear olive or almond oil over them and leave for twelve to twenty-four hours. This should loosen the scales. When you next wash the hair the scales should wash off.
* If the skin under the cradle cap looks inflamed, visit your doctor who can prescribe a cream to rub into the skin.

Infant Remedy Guide

COLDS

Most babies suffer from the snuffles at some stage in the early months. But a healthy baby should be able to recover from a cold in a couple of days. If your baby has a runny nose and is feeding normally and sleeping at night, there is nothing to worry about. However, if she appears to have a chest infection and/or isn't feeding as much as usual, visit your doctor.

Aromatherapy remedy

Put a couple of drops of lavender or pine oil in a vaporiser in your baby's room at night. This may help to clear his or her nose and encourage better sleep.

Practical tips

Keep your baby away from smoky and polluted environments and don't take her out if it is cold and windy. Try breastfeeding more often – the extra fluid will help your baby if she is a little dehydrated.

COLIC

This is a problem faced by many parents in the first few months and usually happens after feeding. A colicky baby will cry and may draw her legs up or stretch them right out as if in pain. The crying may go on for a few hours and often happens in the early evening – just when your partner has got home and wants some time with the baby!

It is thought colic is caused by wind, and produces sharp abdominal pains or cramps, usually lasting until the baby is around three months old. Both breastfed and bottlefed babies can suffer from colic, but there is still disagreement about what colic really is. Colic is sometimes used as a term for a baby who simply cries a lot for no particular reason. Some babies just do cry a great deal and can be inconsolable, so don't feel it is your fault – and this problem does resolve itself naturally when the baby reaches three or four months.

Herbal remedy

Give your baby some dill or fennel seed tea. Simply simmer a teaspoonful of seeds in one pint of water for ten minutes. Then strain and cool and feed to your baby in a bottle or on a plastic spoon. This is a very effective remedy. Or, if you're breastfeeding, try drinking fennel tea on a regular basis. This will pass through to your breastmilk.

Aromatherapy remedy

Try giving your baby a soothing tummy massage using two drops of Roman chamomile oil to 100ml (5tbsp) of almond oil. Or, if your baby is over three months old, mix one drop of Roman chamomile oil with one tablespoonful of milk and drop this mixture into your baby's bath water.

NATURAL BABY CARE

Caution: Never put neat essential oils into your baby's bath.

Practical tips
Always wind your baby after a feed, by sitting her up on your knee or leaning her over your shoulder and gently patting the back. Try giving your baby a bottle of cooled, boiled water if you think she is thirsty rather than hungry. Try and comfort your baby – perhaps by gentle rocking or putting her in a sling and walking around the house. Infacol, available from chemists, is also an effective and gentle medication.

GLUEY EYE
This is a common problem in small babies. It is a mild eye infection caused by blood or fluid getting into your baby's eye during the birth. Your baby's eyelashes may be glued together after sleep and/or she may have pus in the inner corner of the eye.

Homoeopathic remedy
Bathe the eye with Euphrasia or Hypercal tincture. To do this, add two drops of the tincture to an eyebath of cooled, boiled water. If it's difficult using an eyebath, just dip some cotton wool in the mixture and wipe outwards from the inner corner of the eye. Make sure you use a fresh piece of cotton wool for each eye.

Practical tips
Wash your hands before you clean your baby's eyes. You could also try bathing the eyes with cotton wool dipped in cooled, boiled water using the method above. Or, express a little breast milk and drop it into the infected eye – this often works miracles!

TEETHING
Your baby may cut her first tooth at any time during the first year – although the average age is usually five to six months. The

POST-NATAL HEALTH

first tooth is usually in front at the bottom. While some babies have no problems with teething, others may suffer pain from sore swollen gums, as well as having colds, coughs, earache, diarrhoea and sleeplessness. You may be able to see where your baby's gum is sore and red where the tooth is about to come through, or that one cheek is flushed. Your baby may dribble, gnaw and chew on things, but it is sometimes hard to tell whether this is due to teething.

Aromatherapy remedy
Add one or two drops of Roman chamomile oil to a vaporiser or bowl of hot water and place this in your baby's room at night.

Homoeopathic remedy
If your baby has hot and red or pale and cold cheeks or has a red spot on one cheek, and cries out in her sleep, try Chamomilla. This can be bought either as tablets and crushed or in the form of specially prepared teething granules.

Practical tips
Try rubbing your baby's gums with a finger, as the pressure will often help. Give your baby something hard to chew such as a teething ring which can be kept in the fridge (don't keep it in the freezer or it will be too cold) or a piece of cold carrot or celery (stay close to make sure your baby doesn't choke). Try to avoid giving your baby too many doses of medicines or teething gels and avoid rusks because almost all contain some sugar. Even at this stage, constant chewing and sucking on sugary things can cause tooth decay.

THRUSH

This is an infection caused by a yeast which lives in the mouth and intestines. It is usually kept under control by bacteria but it can get out of hand, producing an irritating rash. It will then produce white patches which can be sore and/or itchy. While it isn't serious, it can be common in young babies.

Your baby has oral thrush if you can see white patches on the tongue or the inside of her cheeks. These may look like bits of milk, but won't come off if wiped with a cloth.

Practical tips

Wash your nipples carefully after each breastfeed, as they can become infected. Don't use soap on them – just water. Don't wear breastpads. If you are bottlefeeding, buy a special soft teat and clean it carefully and sterilise after each feed.

GENITAL THRUSH

This can be confused with nappy rash. But the main difference is that thrush usually starts around the anus and spreads outwards, sometimes up to the tummy button, while nappy rash will begin in the baby's creases.

Homoeopathic remedy

Change your baby's nappy frequently and wash her bottom in Hypercal lotion. Then dry well – you could even try using a hairdryer on a low setting.

Practical tips

Don't use bubble baths in your baby's bath and stop using plastic pants over your baby's nappies until the rash has cleared. Let as much fresh air as possible get to your baby's bottom. Also try applying live yoghurt to your baby's bottom to ease itching.

POST-NATAL HEALTH

When to Contact Your Doctor

Always contact your doctor if your baby has any of the following symptoms.

IT'S URGENT IF YOUR BABY

* Has a fit or turns blue or very pale.
* Is particularly drowsy or difficult to wake, or doesn't appear to know you.
* Has quick, difficult or grunting breathing.
* Develops a purple, bruised-looking rash just beneath the surface of the skin, which doesn't go away when you press it.

IT MAY BE SERIOUS IF YOUR BABY

* Has diarrhoea or vomiting.
* Cries for a very long time or in an unusual way or appears to be in pain.
* Is unusually hot or cold or lifeless.
* Has a hoarse cough and is breathing noisily.
* Refuses to eat.
* Screams when exposed to bright lights.

Don't hesitate to contact your doctor immediately, even if you have already seen him or her but your baby isn't getting any better. If you are very worried and a doctor can't get to you quickly enough, take your baby to the accident and emergency department of the nearest hospital with a children's unit.

Coping with Crying

Many newborn babies cry a lot – often to the utter distraction of their parents who simply cannot find a way to soothe them. If you have fed, changed and rocked your baby and she is still crying, try these suggestions:

* Is your baby tired? Some babies will cry when they are exhausted and simply need some sleep. As a new parent, this may seem strange, but putting your fractious baby in her cot can often solve the problem!
* Try carrying your baby around in a sling – the rocking motion will help to soothe her and may even encourage sleep!
* Wrap your baby tightly in a shawl, so the arms and legs are restricted. This often calms a baby down and is very effective for babies up to two months old.
* Take your baby to visit a cranial osteopath. If you had a very long, difficult birth or a forceps delivery, this may have caused tension in your baby, which an osteopath can help to relieve. I highly recommend cranial osteopathy for babies.
* Try playing music that you listened to when you were pregnant – even if it's loud rock music. Its familiarity may pacify your baby.
* Go out! Whether you push your baby in a pram or buggy or drive around in the car with your baby in the back, sometimes just leaving the house will help you both.
* Take all your baby's clothes off and lie her on a mat in a warm room – some babies adore being naked.
* Give your baby a cuddle. Small babies need plenty of affection and loving.
* If your baby always cries after feeding he or she may have colic (see page 82 for solutions).

Caution: Crying can be a sign of illness. If your baby's cry sounds different to normal, or there is something unusual

POST-NATAL HEALTH

about the way your baby is behaving, then contact your doctor immediately.

If your baby's crying gets too much for you:

* Leave her with a friend or relative for an hour just to give yourself a break and to get some rest.
* Put your baby down in a cot or pram and just walk away for a brief while. Make sure your baby is OK, and go into another room or even outdoors. Give it a short amount of time, perhaps five to ten minutes, and then return.
* Get in touch with an organisation which offers support for parents of crying babies. One such group – Cry-SIS – has branches in different areas and will put you in touch with other mothers who have had the same problem (see Useful Addresses).

Glossary

Areola – The darker area surrounding the nipple.

Colostrum – The earliest kind of liquid from a mother's breasts. Your breasts may begin producing it in late pregnancy and it is available for your baby as soon as he or she is born. Colostrum is a yellowish liquid which contains all the antibodies your baby needs to protect him or her from illness and disease. Between two and six days later, your breasts will produce a more mature milk.

Epidural – A local anaesthetic injected into the spine to assist childbirth.

Episiotomy – This is a cut made in the perineum by a midwife or doctor to enlarge the opening during the birth of your baby. It is used if the baby is in distress and needs a rapid delivery, or if your tissues are so tight that either they hold the baby in or there's a risk of your tearing. On balance, it is thought preferable to have a controlled, pain-free cut than an uncontrolled jagged tear which could damage the anus.

Haemoglobin – An oxygen-combining protein carrying iron, present in red blood cells.

Lochia – Bleeding and discharge after the birth.

Mastitis – This is a breast infection, usually caused by a blocked milk duct. You will know if you have mastitis if you have a red patch on a hot tender breast. You may also feel feverish with a temperature and headaches. Mastitis should be

POST-NATAL HEALTH

treated as quickly as possible, or it could result in a breast abscess. Your GP will prescribe a course of antibiotics.

Perineum – The area which surrounds your vagina and between your vagina and anus.

Recti muscles – The muscles which run up the centre of the abdomen. These usually separate during the later stage of pregnancy, and gentle exercise after the birth can bring them back together.

Useful Addresses

Association for Post-natal Illness
25 Jerdan Place
London SW6 1BE
Tel: 0171-386 0868

Caesarean Support Group
81 Elizabeth Way
Cambridge CB4 1BQ
Tel: 01223 314211

Cry-SIS
BM Cry-SIS
London WC1N 3XX
Tel: 0171-404 5011

La Leche League of Great Britain
BM 3424
London WC1N 3XX
Tel: 0171-242 1278 (24-hour answerphone)

Meet-a-Mum Association (MAMA)
14 Willis Road
Croydon
Surrey CR 2XX
Tel: 0181-665 0357

National Childbirth Trust (NCT)
Alexandra House
Oldham Terrace
London W3 6NH
Tel: 0181-992 8637

Accredited Complementary Medicine Practitioners

Send an SAE to any of the following for a list of registered practitioners in your area.

British College of Naturopathy and Osteopathy
Frazer House
6 Netherall Gardens
London NW3 5RR
Tel: 0171-435 8728

The British Homoeopathic Association
27a Devonshire Street
London W1N 1RJ
Tel: 0171-935 2163

The International Federation of Aromatherapists
Stamford House
2–4 Chiswick High Road
London W4 1TH
Tel: 0181- 742 2605

Osteopathic Centre for Children
Suite 4, 1st Floor
19a Cavendish Square
London W1M 9AD
Tel: 0171-495 1231

Index

A
Abdominal exercise 61-62, 64-65
Addresses 91-92
Afterpains 11, 29
Ailments, curing 25-31, 81-85
Alcohol 36
Antidepressants 55-56
Areola 34, 89
Aromatherapy 23-24

B
B, vitamin 21, 57
Baby blues 19-20, 29-30, 51-52
 see also emotions
Backache 25-26, 63, 74-75
Bending 25, 74-75
Birth, difficult 12-14
Body shape 11-12, 16, 61
 see also exercising
Bonding 77
Bottlefeeding 43-45
Breastfeeding 14-16, 33-41, 44-45
 problems 37-41
Breathing exercise 67-68

C
Caesarean birth 10, 14, 28, 61
Care, post-natal 17-19
Colds 81-82
Colic 36, 82-83
Colostrum 15, 89
Constipation 13, 20, 27-28
Contraception 16, 19, 55
Cradle cap 81
Crying baby 86-88
Cut at birth see episiotomy

D
Depression, post-natal 19-20, 29-30, 51-59
Diet, healthy 20-22, 36
Discharge, vaginal see lochia

E
Emotions 10
Engorgement, breast 15, 38
Epidural 25, 74, 89
Episiotomy 11, 19, 26, 27, 89
Exercising 61-75
 see also body shape
Expressing milk 42-43

F
Fatigue 30
Folic acid 22

G
Glossary 89-90
Gluey eye 83

H
Haemoglobin 21, 89

Haemorrhoids 28-29, 63
Hair Loss 17
Homoepathy 24-25

I
Infant ailments 81-85
Insomnia 29
Iron 21

L
Let-down reflex 15, 35
Lifting 74
Linea negra 16
Lochia 12, 89
Lumpy breasts 39

M
Magnesium 57
Massage baby 77-79
Mastitis 39-40, 89-90
Meditation 68
Menstruation 16, 19
Milk duct, blocked 15, 38-40

N
Nappy rash 80-81
Natural remedies 23-31
Neck exercise 69
nipples, sore 37
nursing bra 15

P
Pelvic exercise 62-64, 66, 71
Perineum 11, 13, 27, 63, 90

Piles *see* haemorrhoids
Psychotherapy 56
Puerperal psychosis 53

R
Recipes, weaning 47-48
Recovery tips 13-14
Recti muscles 61, 90
Red patch 39
Relationship with partner 22, 58
Relaxation 67-73

S
Sex life 19, 53
Shoulder exercise 69
Skin 30-31, 79-81
Smoking 36
Solids 45-46
Stitches 26-27

T
Tear at birth *see* episiotomy
Teething 83-84
Thrush 84-85
Tranquillisers 55, 56-57

U
Urinating 11-12, 63

W
Weaning 46-49

Z
Zinc 21-22, 57

HOW TO ORDER YOUR BOXTREE BOOKS BY LIZ EARLE

❏ 0 7522 1699 6	Liz Earle's Bikini Diet	£4.99

Liz Earle's Quick Guides
Available Now

❏ 1 85283 542 7	Aromatherapy	£3.99
❏ 1 85283 544 3	Baby and Toddler Foods	£3.99
❏ 1 85283 543 5	Food Facts	£3.99
❏ 1 85283 546 X	Vegetarian Cookery	£3.99
❏ 0 7522 1619 8	Evening Primrose Oil	£3.99
❏ 0 7533 1614 7	Herbs for Health	£3.99
❏ 1 85283 984 8	Successful Slimming	£3.99
❏ 1 85283 989 9	Vitamins and Minerals	£3.99
❏ 1 85283 979 1	Detox	£3.99
❏ 0 7522 1635 X	Hair Loss	£3.99
❏ 0 7522 1636 8	Youthful Skin	£3.99
❏ 0 7522 1680 5	Healthy Pregnancy	£3.99
❏ 0 7522 1636 8	Dry Skin and Eczema	£3.99
❏ 0 7522 1626 0	Juicing	£3.99
❏ 0 7522 1631 7	Acne	£3.99
❏ 0 7522 1645 7	Beating Cellulite	£3.99
❏ 0 7522 1673 2	Food Combining	£3.99
❏ 0 7522 1675 9	Food Allergies	£3.99
❏ 0 7522 1685 6	Healthy Menopause	£3.99

Coming Soon

❏ 0 7522 1641 4	Cod Liver Oil	£3.99
❏ 0 7522 1668 6	Beating PMS	£3.99
❏ 0 7522 1663 5	Antioxidants	£3.99

ACE Plan Titles

❏ 1 85283 518 4	Liz Earle's Ace Plan The New Guide to Super Vitamins A, C and E	£4.99
❏ 1 85283 554 0	Liz Earle's Ace Plan Weight-Loss for Life	£4.99

All the books shown on the previous page are available at your local bookshop or can be ordered direct from the publisher. Just tick the titles you want and fill in the form below. Prices and availability subject to change without notice.

Boxtree Cash Sales,
PO Box 11, Falmouth, Cornwall TR10 9EN

Please send cheque or postal order for the value of the book(s), and add the following for postage and packing:

UK including BFPO – £1.00 for one book, plus 50p for the second book, and 30p for each additional book ordered up to a £3.00 maximum.

Overseas including Eire – £2.00 for the first book, plus £1.00 for the second book, and 50p for each additional book ordered.

OR
please debit this amount from my Access/VISA card (delete as appropriate)

Card number ☐☐☐☐☐☐☐☐☐☐☐☐☐☐☐☐☐☐☐

Amount £ ....

Expiry date on card ....

Signed ....

Name ....

Address ....

....

....